Jade Chi Do ®

A Practice Unifying
Stillness and Movement

by

Dwayne T. Feeley

I dedicate this book to those who are on the path of discovery, who intuitively feel a sort of silent calling - a knowing from deep within that they are more than the limits they may presently have - and who know it is time to cast their pebble upon the water so that its ripples will be felt around the world.

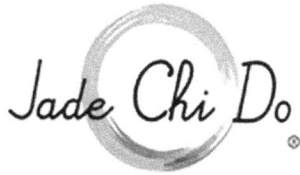

Jade Chi Do

AUTHOR'S NOTE
In The Realm Of All Possibilities

In the late 1990s, I traveled to Boston to attend a symposium of doctors speaking on alternative health and exercise protocols. I don't remember much other than one oncology speaker. His speech to his colleagues and members of the public who were in attendance has stayed with me all these years.

He said that he noticed people under a doctor's care often had their confidence broken by their doctor or someone else with authority and influence, which negatively affected their health results. Whether a conventional or alternative doctor, the detrimental result of a poorly delivered opinion was the same.

He said to his colleagues on the podium that the placebo in many drug trials showed minimal improvement from the baseline, and in many cases, was just under or above the chemical being tested. (For readers who are unfamiliar with placebos, it is a substance that has no therapeutic effect, and is used for comparison purposes when a new drug is being tested.)

He concluded by saying, "If something is helping or even working more effectively, why would I want to influence them with my opinion and take that away? I know there are many of you that may disagree, but I ask you to think about this before you pass judgment on those under your care."

That statement rings as loud and clear in my memory today as it did when I first heard it over twenty years ago. Today, after having so much time to meditate on the wisdom of those words, I am more certain than ever that it is not the mere word "belief" that makes us whole again, or that helps us surpass our own previous limits, but its root, which is found in our deepest, innermost confidence.

I won't bore you with case studies and scientific data. You can easily find that if you'd like to do some research on your own. I want to go one step further by showing you how to become extraordinary at your own highest level.

You always have a choice between cynicism and growth, between poking holes in new information or following a recipe that will help you discover that which has been patiently waiting within you for you to discover and use.

When barriers are first broken, such as the four-minute mile, resisting extreme cold, or other feats that were previously considered medically or physically impossible, and when many others break those same barriers shortly afterward because they have been made aware that the barrier was in fact artificial, does it not reveal the truth that you are capable of much more than you know?

In this book, I will share something that is close to my heart; something I've known from personal experience for decades but have been afraid to reveal for fear of being ridiculed by those who don't understand these teachings. However, I know now that the time has come for me to put my own ego aside for the benefit of others.

Dedicated practice to the recipe given in these pages will build true, innermost confidence and other extraordinary possibilities that are available to those who are willing to expand beyond what they have been told is impossible.

A Note on Science

In earlier centuries, anything that was extremely out of the ordinary was considered to be mystical and supernatural. But as science caught up, many of these superstitious misconceptions left the realm of mystery and became demonstrable, scientific facts.

However, this is not to say science has turned over every stone and explained every mystery. There are many that are still unexplored, or simply outside the realm of scientific exploration. If you were able to talk to a caveman and describe a lighter that gives a flame on demand, or even a matchstick, he would think it impossible until you showed him. Likewise, if you showed a mobile phone playing a movie to someone in Salem, Massachusetts, during the witch trials, that might not end well for you.

But modern science is catching up quickly. We are evolving faster than ever before as one discovery reveals another. Most who discover untapped human abilities sound the trumpet, hoping to achieve fame and fortune by breaking a four-minute-mile kind of barrier of their own. I am not here to sound any trumpets. There are enough doing that. I am simply saying that it's time we come forward and become examples to those who would see us as different, and to carry the light to those who have not yet experienced or even imagined it.

Can you imagine if five hundred people broke the four-minute-mile or any other perceived barrier at the same time? This would indeed create a bigger ripple effect and extend the limits of our collective paradigm.

This book has a simple goal - to lower your blinders so that you can begin to see that which has always been awaiting discovery within you. It will take courage and gumption, like every great explorer who came before you, but the rewards will be incalculable. If you choose to accept this mission, read on. Be sure to read the special story after the initial training. I feel it will be a great complement to what I am sharing with you. If you feel overwhelmed or confused by the lessons in part one, you can start with the story in part two and return to the lessons later.

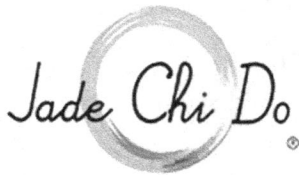

Jade Chi Do

FOREWORD

Words like "groundbreaking" and "revolutionary" are used so often these days, they have become meaningless, so I don't expect you to believe me when I say that this book is both, but it is.

I make my living as a producer and screenwriter but I started out as a copy editor. I still edit, but only when I'm inspired by the subject matter and the author, and that is certainly the case here, on both counts. There are thousands of self-help books on the market, but it is rare to encounter books that are truly transformative. That is, a book that both motivates the reader and provides the step-by-step (and surprisingly simple) tools to become an advanced student of the discipline being taught.

As the saying goes, when the mind is ready, a teacher appears. Therefore, the exercises and meditations described in this book must be performed with sincerity and patience. The question is, are you ready?

If you are, you have just found a master very much like the masters of ancient times who taught students with movements and visualizations handed down through countless generations which were designed to unlock powers and abilities that gave devotees other-worldly skills – skills that could be applied not only to combat but to all areas of their lives. As an old adage says, one who has mastered a discipline will display it in their every action.

You will find that the exercises in this book are deceptively simple. They require no special strength or skill. Anyone can do them. But when practiced whole-heartedly, abilities and ways of seeing that are uncommon in the modern world will be unleashed. You will recognize these abilities because they have always existed within you. It is what Dwayne calls the "warm life force". You have encountered it before, though you may not know you have; for instance, moments when you felt you were being watched and turned to discover that you were, or when you performed some action unthinkingly but with absolute perfection. Athletes call it "the zone" – a place they enter when they are performing at their highest level that has an almost mystical feeling. The good news is that feeling is available to everyone, not just professional athletes, and it can be applied to anything – sports, art, business, even relationships.

This is not just another book to get you pumped up with positive platitudes, it is a treasure trove of specific exercises and meditations that will feel very mysterious at first but will quickly come to feel very familiar, reacquainting you with a deeper knowing you have always possessed but didn't know how to discover, develop, and use . . . until now. Think of a dragon that has been sleeping for years – a dragon you are about to awaken – and the dragon is YOU.

Again, don't let the simplicity of the exercises and visualizations in this book fool you. You are about to tap into a dormant superpower that will change your life forever. It's a scientific fact that every human being – except for those fortunate few the world refers to as geniuses – use less than ten percent of their brains. What a waste. Jade Chi Do is not supernatural, or some ungodly dark art. It's simply making full use of a significant portion of the rest of that "gray matter" that has been dormant within you all these years. You are about to activate it. Put on your seatbelt and hold on to your hat. A great adventure awaits you – an adventure within.

Mark Rickerby

Owner, Temple Gate Films

TV Series Creator, Producer, Screenwriter

Over 25 Chicken Soup for the Soul contributions

Black Belt Magazine

InsideKungFu Magazine

TABLE OF CONTENTS

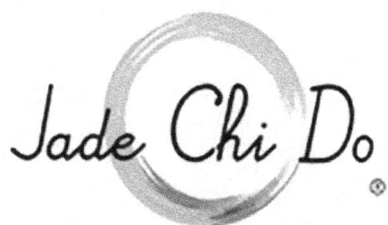

Jade Chi Do

PART I

The Way of Jade Chi Do

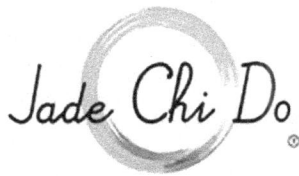

Jade Chi Do

PREFACE

This is a true story. My message has been burning within me, waiting to be released for years, but the moment never felt right. It still doesn't, but I can't hold this message inside any longer. Actually, I'm nervous about releasing this information to the world. I don't want to be rejected or ridiculed, but I know I must put myself aside. My life has been forged by many factors, not all of which were ordinary. However, when combined and looked at together, I'm sure you will agree that they are extremely out of the ordinary.

When I was very young, I ended up living on the streets and was taken in by a Kung Fu master. I was allowed to stay in the school and sleep on the floor as long as I cleaned the school and toilet. Later, I became a student instructor and taught for him. In exchange for this work, he shared much with me.

I also worked for my teacher as a security person at concerts. We traveled with bands from venue to venue in a little van. I worked backstage and in front of the stage where scaffolding was laid out to keep fans away from the performers. I protected AC/DC and many other popular bands of that time. I met David Lee Roth when he was still with Van Halen. My main job was to stop fans who managed to get past the scaffolding.

When I spent those younger days with my teacher, I had no idea how much wisdom he was transferring to me, and often didn't understand the meaning of his words and actions until much later. I will write more about this part of my past in a future book, and some in a coming chapter.

I eventually moved out of the school. I was making friends and having fun. I was training with a friend one day when he broke his leg. The first thing he said was, "I don't want to lose my job." He worked at the fish market filleting fish. So I said, "I guess I'm going to be a fish cutter."

I had never filleted a fish in my life but I managed to cut one ton per day with another cutter. Once my friend was healed, I stopped and he went back. I didn't expect to enjoy that work so much. There was something very satisfying about it. It was hard giving it up but it felt good to know that I helped my friend keep his job.

I was in my late teens at this point, training hard to compete in a tournament in China. I was good with many weapons and forms, but my plans were derailed by another life-changing event. I was exercising on a trampoline in the backyard of a house where I was renting a room. About one hundred feet away, another young man was hitting marbles with the thick end of a two-section pool cue. I finished my exercise and was jumping down from the trampoline, but before my feet hit the ground, something very hard hit me in the head. I landed on my feet in a natural fighting stance out of instinct, thinking someone had hit me intentionally, but nobody was close to me. I looked around to see what had hit me and saw the pool cue on the ground nearby. I later learned that it had slipped out of his hand and flew backward like bats sometimes do in baseball games. The odds of hitting me from a hundred feet away while I was in mid-air were astronomical, but it happened.

I felt alright as I walked into the house and sat in a chair, but then I started to see a sort of white static; black and white dots, like watching an old TV set with no signal. I knew something was not right so I went to the hospital, and as we walked in, a college intern took me to get an X-ray. After he examined the X-ray, he said, "Nothing is broken. You can go home, but don't sleep, and watch for any unusual symptoms."

I went home and laid on my bunk. The pain in my head was immense, but every once in a while, there would be a fraction of a second when there was no pain at all. It came and went like clockwork, moments of relief amid constant agony. Then I started hearing a voice like a coach that kept saying, "Use the memory of the moments when there was no pain, and focus on that."

I lay there for a few hours just doing that, living the memory, and every time the painless moments came, they got longer and longer. It was working! Then something changed. It's hard to explain, but I started to get a cold feeling at the tips of my toes and fingers. There was nothing different visually, but I remember thinking that this feeling had a color, and it was black. I felt it slowly move up my arms and legs like a slithering snake, and as it got close to my shoulders, someone screamed "Push!" at me from inside. At that moment, I felt a white light push back to the tips of my fingers and toes. This went back and forth for about an hour. I continued to remember the painless, in-between times, trying to calm my mind and stretch that moment out longer each time.

I decided there must be something else wrong with me. I was taken back to the hospital. As we walked in, just moving was tremendously difficult for me. Ironically, the head neurosurgeon was walking into the hospital at that moment. It was perfect timing. He was walking next to me when he looked at me and said, "Have you been seen yet?"

I said yes. Then he asked, "Have you had a CT scan?"

I told him I hadn't. (In the early 1980's, X-rays were more common.) The doctor rushed me in to get the CT scan. He looked at the results, said "Oh, my God", then rushed me to surgery. The first X-ray had shown nothing because it was a circle of crushed bone that was hard to see, but the doctor spotted it.

I was near death as the doctor rushed me into surgery. I died on the table. I remember lights and such, a third-person view. It was like I was over my body, looking down on them operating on me, then there was just white light. There's more to that story, but it's not important now. Later, I woke up with stitches across my entire forehead. I looked like Frankenstein's monster. The fear of dying I felt before the surgery was completely gone. Then (and I cringe telling you this), I started to do headstand push-ups. As I mentioned, I was trying to go to China to

4

compete in a Kung Fu tournament. I was obsessed with training and would often exercise at random times like this, but this was the worst possible time not only to exercise, but to do this particular exercise, since I wasn't supposed to have any pressure in my head immediately after skull surgery. Perhaps in my drugged state, I didn't realize how bad my condition really was.

Forty-eight hours after the surgery, the doctor came in and pushed on my head where the hole was. He seemed confused at first, then shocked, then amazed. He removed the many stitches and added two words to his final report – "Miraculous healing."

Mind you, I had never healed that quickly before, and it hasn't happened again since. (Then again, I haven't been hit by any pool cues lately, either.) A unique awareness that I've had since birth became much stronger after this event. It has not stopped me from making poor decisions, but I now learn from my mistakes, and strive to do better. It is this awareness I hope to impart to you in this book. It is not just something that will help you stop forgetting your keys or find the remote control for the TV, it is a force that can give you abilities very few possess, and transform your life and how you see the world around you. Wonders await you in the pages and years ahead.

A few years later, I met a woman through a band I was in and fell in love with her. She had two wonderful young children. We got married and they became my stepsons. I loved them both, and as far as I'm concerned, they will always be my sons. But for some reason, I connected more deeply with the older of the two. He and I hit it off immediately.

He loved to help me when I was working around the house. I was chopping wood one day and he was stacking it in a wooden box in the back of my old Chevy truck. If a small piece of wood broke off, he would pick it up, put a wedge in any split he could find, and hit it with a sledgehammer to break it apart. He was ten years old at the time.

I was on the ground splitting wood while he played in the back of the truck when I heard him scream. I turned to look and saw him holding his right leg. I ran over, pulled his pant leg up, and saw some blood and his bone poking out in the middle of his shin. I had a strangely fast, instinctive reaction to put my right hand over it. When I did, there was a bright flash, then a weird, painful feeling from my heart to my palm. It's hard to explain. It happened so quickly and I was so panicked, I didn't pay attention. I jumped down to get behind the wheel of my truck and take him to the hospital, but as I did, I heard him quietly say, "Dad, what are you doing?"

I turned back to him and said, "Your leg!"

He answered, "Dad, what happened? It's okay now."

I looked at his leg again and there was nothing wrong with it. I truly cried with relief, but also confusion. I never questioned that day, and nothing like that has happened since.

In the 1990's, I was driving my Jeep Cherokee to meet my workers to take them to an emergency job for my company. It was late in the day and almost dark. I wasn't wearing my seatbelt - a bad habit of mine in those days. I was driving fast because of the emergency situation at the job when another very strange thing happened. It gives me chills to write about it now, but at the time, it seemed like nothing As I was driving, a voice from behind me shouted, "Dwayne, put your seatbelt on!" I jumped a bit and brushed it off. (And no, I do not hear voices all the time, and I am not crazy. Fear of people thinking that is one reason I have been so hesitant to tell my story for so long.)

I was driving along, confused and a little scared, when the voice shouted the same words again. It was so clear and loud, it was as if someone was sitting right behind me. I thought to myself "what the heck" and put the seatbelt on just so whoever it was would stop yelling.

Less than two miles ahead, the road changed from pavement to dirt at a sharp curve. I wasn't speeding but I had to swerve to avoid running over something that was laying in the road, and when I did, I drove my Jeep right off the edge. I was hurtling off the road with a small drop-off and then trees. I was certain that my number was up when the Jeep came to a sudden stop. I had been thrown around a little but when I lifted my head again, I was horrified to see that the windshield had been blown out. One would think it was caused by simple inertia, but then I looked to my right and saw that the passenger seat was gone too, and the bolts that held the seat had been completely pulled out of the floorboard. I looked behind my seat and saw that the double-wide back seat had also broken free of the floor, bolts and all, and was leaning forward. Then I noticed that the back window had also been blown out and fallen into the cab!

I looked back down at myself, still in my seatbelt, and wondered why the bolts to my seat had held on. Without the seatbelt I had been "ordered" to fasten, I would surely have been a human catapult.

When I got out, I looked under the Jeep and saw that it had been stopped by a tree stump that was the perfect height to catch the axle, which stopped the Jeep dead in its tracks. If it had kept going, I would not have survived. At the time, all I thought of was that voice. Later, I thought I had imagined it and it was just dumb luck. But in retrospect, I have to ask why I was apparently protected again.

Many other odd things started to happen after that. Some uncommon abilities that I always had started to peak. I started teaching a little but felt that my ego was getting the best of me. Though I didn't understand these occurrences, I had the feeling that I was being given a message of some kind, a message I should share with the world, but I pushed it aside out of fear of being ridiculed. I had written a small book when I was younger but kept it a secret. I have imperfections like anyone else, so there was probably some self-doubt too. Who was I to be chosen to deliver a message from another world?

My Ego Buster

Later, our family house burned down. We were not well insured so it was hard to manage even our basic needs for a while. About ten days later, I brought my wife to the doctor for a severe backache. A few days later, she was diagnosed with leukemia; and fifteen months after that, she passed away in my arms. One of the hardest things I've ever had to do was call our eldest son and tell him that his mom had passed away. She was only thirty-six. Even now, I choke up thinking about it.

The moment she died, I held her head with my right hand. She told me she loved me with her last breath. The very second she passed, I had a feeling like thousands of lightning bolts in the hand that was behind her head, like something flowing or passing through my hand. Then there was only darkness around her body. Nothing out of the ordinary had happened before that moment so I was not expecting such an intense experience.

Losing my wife devastated and humbled me so much, I lost much of the desire to share any message. But the story kept unfolding anyway, with or without my agreement or acceptance. I had a feeling of becoming something, like a caterpillar emerging from a cocoon, from darkness to light, but I couldn't understand it myself so how could I explain it to others? The message I felt years ago, and repeatedly throughout the years, was staring me right in the face again during the saddest event of my life. But the sadness caused me to pack it away again in some deep corner of my mind, or so I thought.

I continued to encounter challenges, many of which were self-induced because I never wanted to listen to others who might have helped me. Every year, the message would bubble up and I would push it away. I tried to decipher and capture the message in writing again in 2013 but because of insecurities about my imperfections, and fear of rejection, I pushed it away and stayed in limbo.

Now here I am, twenty years since I first became aware of this phenomenon, still feeling pressure to release the message and maybe even shift the paradigm we're all living under right now. It's like a soda bottle being shaken, building up pressure within. The voice from inside me is the same one I heard when I was young and in so much pain decades ago.

But I am finally putting pen to paper, the words like a net thrown to capture whatever these events and powers might mean. I have had more problems running from the pressure than I can imagine I will have by trying to communicate the right words.

I see people everywhere in the world reaching, knowing there is something out there, but only finding more confusion. Still, I ask, is it finally time? I feel it is and that we are in a time of quickening. I believe it is time to evolve, but whether it is or not, I am taking the proverbial leap of faith and delivering this message, like a child playing hide-and-seek and yelling, "Ready or not, here I come!" If I only help one other person, and that person helps another, and so on - the waves will be felt across the world. At the very least, I will have finally gotten this story out of my system.

When my late wife and I were first married, we were going on our honeymoon when we both agreed that it didn't feel right to leave the boys. Funds were too tight anyway, so we turned the car around and went back home. We decided to take a short honeymoon and vacation the next year when I made more money. I worked with a small company making water wells. Each year, I said, "Next year, we will have more, but nine years passed and "next year" never came.

This saddens me even now, but this is also why I must not wait. Everything within me screams "it is time." I must put my fears behind me, learn from my mistakes, and allow that which would have stopped me before to propel me forward now. Again, I believe humanity is experiencing a quickening, and the time is upon not only me, but all of us.

Have you ever had a mysterious experience or feeling and knew there was more to it, but dismissed it as mere intuition? Have you found yourself immersed in your spirituality, whether it be your faith, meditation, or other pursuits, and yet still felt a kind of knowing – a certainty – that there is more that you are not accessing?

My message, if received with an open mind, will indeed remove the blinders we all acquire early in life, placed on us by others, and which we still unknowingly wear.

Whatever has drawn you to be in this moment, reading this message, it is finally time to open up that which has been waiting within. Each chapter in this book is another step that will build your confidence, and as your confidence builds, so will the effectiveness of the message.

The book's goal is to install a specific foundation of confidence, like a ladder, continually ascending to the next step.

I seek not to change your faith or whatever belief system you follow, but only to enhance. Even though you may find similarities, I ask that you keep an open mind. A full cup has no room for more.

You perceive the world around you from your own individual perspective. Therefore, the following chapters will seek to expand your perspective. By achieving this, you will break the chains and gain the ability to accept the message. Part of the message is that you are more than you think – or perceive – you are. In life, we are always discovering how much we don't know, also known as learning. I know this is a bold statement, but you are about to discover that in the biggest way possible. Too many of us are like the man who spent his life in poverty only to discover he had a precious gem in his pocket all along that would have made him wealthy if he knew it was there. In the following pages, I hope to help you find the gem hidden inside you, and in so doing, change your destiny to whatever you want it to be.

Jade Chi Do
®

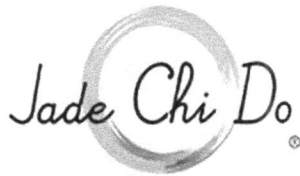

PART I - CHAPTER 1

Awakened Awareness And Healing Through Active Motion Meditation

I n this book, I will be teaching a new and unique art called Jade Chi Do. It is unlike anything you have ever experienced. If you follow the instructions contained here and dedicate yourself to the exercises, you will develop a level of internal energy (chi) that has been attained by only a very few masters. You won't have to wait years. Through dedication, the gifts become tangible, growing every step of the way. The extraordinary will become ordinary.

Before you write this off as exaggeration, let me tell you something you have probably already noticed - again, there is a quickening happening around the world, an inner knowing sweeping through humanity that the human mind is capable of much more, and that these abilities are accessible to everyone, not just gurus, sages, masters, and monks. Science is increasingly supporting this idea. However, as with every area of higher learning, the key to unlocking this untapped potential is finding someone who can translate and communicate it; someone who can help you remove the blockages between who you are and who you want to be; between what you think your mind is capable of and what it is truly capable of. If I were asked to draw an analogy of this process, it would be of dynamiting a cave to release people trapped in darkness; giving them their first view of the great, pitching, swirling universe. The magnitude of this practice is that big.

What is Jade Chi Do?

The simplest way to describe it is "a new form of active motion meditation". I know, anticlimactic, right? In fact, you may be thinking, *What? Another meditation technique?* Well, stick with me for a while. Your mind is about to be blown open.

I will be teaching this from the beginning, step-by-step, the same way I learned it. This way, I will be able to convey a tangible vibration, or frequency, to gradually create a sense of control and power within you and over your life, the likes of which you may have never dreamed possible.

Each lesson is a building block to the next. If one becomes impatient and jumps ahead, they will only defeat themselves and limit their ultimate achievement. Active practitioners will learn more quickly and achieve greater results.

Prepare yourself for a great and rewarding journey. Please keep in mind that true success is not a destination but a journey, and the journey is what defines us. The process, not the product.

Have you been trying to find an edge; a quality that can separate you from the crowd? Have you ever experienced actions or reflexes that started before the need for them even became apparent? It could be something as simple as catching a falling cup of coffee without spilling it and having everyone look at you like you're some kind of ninja, to getting a bad feeling in a public place just before something crazy happens. It is this innate ability I want to help you explore and develop in the following pages.

As you read, you will come to realize that this is not a new subject for you. You've always known your mind was capable of much more. Perhaps you've received hint after hint of its abilities, but could never capture or define it. It's not a physical object you can pick up and examine. What people refer to as intuition or a "sixth sense" is intangible. Those who have it don't know how or where to begin to explore it, so most spend their lives mystified, amused, perhaps even confused about the experiences in their lives that are too coincidental to be accidental.

This book is what you have needed all along, like finding a key to an old chest, the contents of which you have always been curious about, but that was too thick and strong to break open. What you are about to read will give you a chance to finally complete what you have always known. There is nothing to lose and a world to gain, and the only thing required of you is an open mind.

A few requests . . .

As I have stated earlier, for best results, take your time reading this book. What one may assume is a simple truth may indeed be something much more. Don't race ahead to the next word or sentence. You have heard the expression "live in the moment". Well, I'm asking you to read in the moment, with no reinterpretation, no comparing to what you already know, as if you were a child again, too young to have any cemented opinions yet. You can allow your analytical, and perhaps cynical, adult mind to take over when you are finished with the book. Then you can accept it as the greatest gift you've ever received, or total hogwash. The choice, of course, is always yours. But skepticism every step of the way may prevent you from receiving all that will be given to you here.

With that, welcome, and read on! You are about to have an experience like no other, and receive something truly unique. I will show you an exercise called Heaven and Earth and ask that you practice it as you read. But in this chapter, we must also work on our connection and communication with our mind and body.

Now let's begin this new journey.

Here are the ground rules for achieving the greatest reward in this practice. It applies to all things that can be learned, but even more so here:

If you find the first few chapters challenging and a little confusing, as your teacher as you travel through this book, I ask that you simply follow along as best you can. And don't worry - you don't need to fully comprehend everything immediately. Like the abilities you will discover within yourself through the faithful practice of the exercises and meditations contained here, awareness sometimes comes slowly. However, your innate, untapped abilities can also be uncovered quickly depending on your level of readiness to receive them, and your dedication to your practice.

I am condensing many years of teaching into these pages. Therefore, in later chapters, I will hasten your learning in a very powerful way - through a story, just as the elders did around the campfire long, long ago.

If you make a choice to learn a new art, it is imperative that you first empty your mind of what you think you already know. Comparison dilutes and distracts from the essence of the new ideas being taught, the same way comparing our experiences today to similar experiences in the past dilutes the present.

"Each morning when I awake, like a scholar at his first class, I prepare a blank mind for the day to write upon." (Circle of Iron, 1978)

There is an old story about a student who sought a martial arts master. He inquired about what he might learn from him, but the master couldn't answer because the student kept talking about his past experiences, hoping to impress the teacher with his knowledge. As he was speaking, the master interrupted him to ask if he would like some tea. The student accepted and continued talking. The master set two cups down and began to pour until the student's cup overflowed and ran all over the table. The student finally stopped talking and said, "The cup is full!" The master smiled and said, "Your mind is like this cup. It is already full of your own opinions. Before I can teach you anything, you must first empty your cup."

Likewise, the depth of your understanding - in fact your ability to learn - will be hampered if you relate and compare new information to what you already know. It's another form of not "living in the now"; that is, conceptualizing our experiences rather than savoring every moment as unique. ("Wow! This is a great sunset, but not as great as that one in Italy last year.")

By comparing, you only reaffirm what you already know. Everyone says they want to learn new things, but most spend lifetimes reaffirming and reiterating the same ideas. This is not growth, it's stagnation. It's a challenge we all face. Everyone is limited by this tendency to one degree or another.

Teachers choose and utilize the method that best enables them to instill the knowledge and abilities their students desire to learn. The speed of this learning can be quick or slow. Art students become proficient in an art by using techniques and movements that may seem basic but are actually engineered to become the building blocks of higher learning and ability. Practicing scales can seem boring and tedious, but it enables the student to someday become a virtuoso.

At risk of overstating this, listening with an open mind and a deep willingness to learn is vastly different from performing actions while only mentally reaffirming what you already know. It is what you do not know that is important, and why you are here.

In our first lesson, we will lay down the building blocks by helping to guide your thoughts through this process, which will maximize your results later.

Let's begin with the idea of discipline. There are many ways to feel rewarded for discipline. In school, we study hard to get good grades. In our occupations as adults, we work and get paid. Our children receive trophies for sports, and certificates for scholastic achievements. Thus, we are hardwired from an early age to associate work with a reward, and to seek those rewards.

One of the hardest things to teach children is delaying gratification. When they want ice cream, they let you know in no uncertain terms that they want it right now, not after they eat their dinner or do a chore. In fact, if you delay a reward, a greater reward often comes later. Granted, this is not always true, but let's look at an example to illustrate this theory.

I love pizza (who doesn't?), but if I gorge myself on it every day, I may start to feel sick. The more pizza I eat, the worse I'll feel. Even if I tell myself I'm going to give it up entirely, once I start to feel better, I forget the discomfort I felt earlier (and the guilt of throwing my diet out the window) and find myself on the phone ordering an extra-large pizza with everything on it. If this happens enough times to make me angry at myself for my lack of discipline, I may resolve to eat pizza every other day instead of every day. (I mean, let's not get crazy!) I might not get sick anymore, but the long-term effects to my appearance (weight gain), my mind (guilt and shame over my lack of willpower), and even my general health (heart disease, etc.) may be significant.

The alternative is knowing that if we make a healthy choice - even if it feels like a sacrifice at first - we will find out later that we will achieve more. Like putting in the time to learn a new skill - the immediate rewards are intangible but every bit as valuable as money or trophies (or ice cream.) The first payment that comes with learning – with slowing our minds and studying the fundamentals - is the virtue of patience. While our reward, for instance, for learning how to play the piano like Beethoven (or Jerry Lee Lewis, whomever you prefer) will not come until later, our journey to reach that end goal is also rewarding as we see ourselves becoming better and more proficient.

In other words, there is pride all along the way, not just at the end. Are we not as strengthened by the climb up the mountain as we are by the victory of reaching its peak? If we stop, or turn around and head backward, we will never see the view from the top; we will never achieve our reward.

So the first step toward learning Jade Chi Do, or anything else, is to start living each day with this kind of discipline; with the knowledge that confusion is the doorway to a higher level of understanding and ability. There's no way around confusion and frustration when learning something new, so we might as well embrace it.

Along with hard work, many people also tend to avoid boredom. But it is also a gift because it means you have learned the material. Boredom is actually a step above confusion!

Now, I'm not saying go become a monk and deny all earthly pleasures, but I am saying that you will be rewarded by committing yourself to this particular discipline, both along the way and when you arrive. The rewards are internal (pride, confidence, inner peace) or external (better health and appearance, success). To achieve the best results, you must constantly develop this discipline as you work toward your goals.

I'm sure you've heard the quote by Mother Teresa "Be the change you want to see in the world." It would be just as true if she advised us to be the change we want to see in our families, workplaces, relationships, even traffic. Be the brave one; the unreasonably happy one, the one who inspires others to be happy; the one who is just as happy after the party as he was when it was happening; the one who acts out of his/her higher self, not his lower one. If you really want to stand out and inspire others, especially those whom you love, you must develop the discipline to rise above all the petty squabbling of life. This ability gives you an almost godlike status, particularly to those who can't resist becoming embroiled in all the mayhem. It's the difference between yelling at other drivers and jockeying for position, or staying in the slow lane (because you left early) and letting the world swirl around you. Let them get high blood pressure while you enjoy the radio and sing your favorite songs.

My point is, when you achieve better physical and emotional health, you can help your family do the same. There's no better and more inspiring teacher than example. Achieving more yourself will enable you to help others achieve more. This is a true win/win for you because you can find the greatest satisfaction and gratification, mentally and physically, from helping others. There is a reason people say internal rewards are more valuable than money. I'm sure you've heard the expression "money can't buy happiness." It's true. Some of the happiest people I've met have been poor, and some of the unhappiest have been rich.

True wealth – that is, internal riches - or at least the potential for it, is already within you, and it's a party that is eternal (and impervious to economic downturns.) If you're not happy before you get to your dream destination (goal), it's very unlikely that you'll be happy when you do. The dye will be cast. Many achieve their dreams, then realize the joy was in the striving and growing. This is why successful actors and billionaires commit suicide, while poor people shake their heads and ask, "Why would he/she do that? He had everything." Obviously not.

Let's change directions for a moment. Another kind of discipline that will help you get to where you want to go is developing a stronger connection to that part of yourself that always wants to help you, the part that is always listening and is usually silent until your "self-talk" becomes too negative, then it jumps in and says, "No! You've worked too hard and been through too much to talk to yourself like that." Have you ever had that kind of argument in your mind, like there are two versions of yourself struggling for dominance? Everyone does.

That little voice is there for you in simpler ways too. For example, have you ever woken up five or ten minutes before your alarm clock was set to ring? You didn't stay up all night watching your clock, yet you woke up at almost exactly the right time. So, since you were asleep, what was actually monitoring the time? There is something inside you that is working even when you're unaware of it. I was told when I was young – I can't remember where – that Native American hunters (who don't have alarm clocks) tap their pillows six times if they want to wake up at six a.m., seven times for seven a.m., etc. They are not only aware of this subconscious ability – this thought that exists outside of their known thought – they depend on it as much as we depend on our iPhone alarm clocks.

I do not wish to compile all of this into one big group called subconscious. For this exercise, the idea is simply to open your mind to a deeper way of thinking, or more accurately, understanding.

Looking at it from another perspective, let's accept that there's a part of our minds that wishes to reward us, and another part that wants to protect us. If speaking in public is scary to someone, that part of their mind will try to protect them by reinforcing reasons why they shouldn't do it. It doesn't know the difference. It doesn't know that public speaking can be incredibly pleasurable and exhilarating. It only understands what hurts or frightens you, maybe more than you do. So it steers you away from what you fear for your own protection, the same way it would a bear or alligator.

So let us create clear and defined thoughts; thoughts that you choose; thoughts that will reward and serve you.

I will go one step further. This part of us that strives to help is also the part that connects us to the intangible. Many say this is where you put your emotions and intentions, and it rewards you for this. But instead of saying you're going to put it out into the universe and it will manifest in you, we are going to dive into the nuts and bolts of what manifestation really is - because that is the wheel we can create. That is the connection that strives to help us and our current bodies here on this earth. You will find that you are rewarded not only in one way or another, but in your whole self, and your evolution will be phenomenal.

What better time to put this to the test than right here and now?

Lesson One: I do not seek belief, I seek confidence.

The first step is easy because all you need to do is follow your instructor. However, easy does not mean unimportant. Remember that the foundation you build now will later support everything that stands upon it. We're going to use our imagination and focus, and our entire bodies.

You've probably heard of several different types of meditations. Maybe you've even tried some of them. Most of them achieve great results. But what we are going to do now is different. We are going to communicate with that part of ourselves that wants to serve us, and this path will be quite rewarding.

For lesson one, again, all you need to do is simply follow my instructions. We're going to connect your breath to your movements in a different way. In some kinds of meditation, you monitor your breath, or a set number of words. Even though you're not thinking anything, you are focusing on your breathing, or on what some people call a mantra.

We are going to do something very different. We are going to get down to the fundamentals and build from there to be able to communicate and discover that part of us waiting to be discovered. This part has expressed itself to you in small ways for many years. Let's see where this training brings us.

I remember a story with Four Blind Men and an Elephant. I heard it as a child so my retelling may not be perfect but the point will be clear. Four blind men were asked to approach an elephant, touch it and say what they thought it was. The elephant was standing still.

The first blind man walked up to the tail, felt it, came back and said the elephant was a hanging vine or a whip and to watch out for it. The second went to his massive leg and said the elephant was an immovable column. The third walked up to the ivory tusk and said the elephant was a spear. The fourth blind man walked up to the elephant's trunk and said the elephant was a large snake that could wrap itself around them.

My point is we may only see parts of something greater within ourselves but not the whole picture. Like the blind men, there is more within you than you know, riches just waiting to be discovered. All that is required is that you allow yourself to learn how to open the window to see more than the part you may feel now.

It is time to begin to lift your own personal blinders so you can create clearer communication with that unknown part of yourself. This part has been revealing itself each day, but like the elephant in the story, you may have been able to define only that which you perceived, dismissing the rest.

Let's now build from the first step.

You are going to observe something in your body that is quite phenomenal, but to do so, you're going to need to let your imagination take control. Some of the greatest things I've seen happen on this earth were a result of people activating this discipline in extreme ways. I've seen people dance with snakes. I've even heard of some people overcoming poison.

I am neither making this up nor advocating these practices. I'm simply saying that I've seen people do some fantastic things. Some of them said they were able to access these abilities because they went into a trance. Accessing that part of us that wants to help is the key. But right now, to be clear, our goals should be a calmer connection, and a mind that is more open to possibilities.

Meditate on this idea: Once a true possibility reveals itself, then the confidence of it happening becomes reality.

With that in mind, let's begin. This exercise is called **The Standing Tree.**

- Stand upright with ample room around you, feet shoulder-width apart, and your hands by your sides.

- Now focus on your breath. (Here's where the imagination part comes in.)

- This is going to sound strange, but allow your hands to become part of your breath, as if you are breathing out of your hands only, or as if your hands are vacuum cleaners.

- Raise your hands upward at your sides until they're above your head, with palms facing the sky, fingers almost touching, as if you're holding a pizza pan on your palms. Keep them limp and relaxed, with your fingers apart, moving your arms and hands like a paintbrush, dragging your hands upward.

- As you are releasing your breath, lower your arms and hands in the same motion, to the sides of your body.

- Repeat slowly upward and downward, breathing slowly. As you lower your hands, you'll feel a gentle sensation, like you're putting your hands through a thick cloud of fog. Just keep your mind clear. Allow your mind to draw in the energy of life, not passively but powerfully. You're sucking life up through the vacuums of your arms. Just breathe in; never mind any visuals. As you are raising your hands and breathing in, you'll start to have different feelings in your hands. Allow this to happen. Don't block anything.

- This exercise is very important because you can learn and feel this particular vibration through this training if you accept the feeling. I know from experience that this works quite well.

I'd like to elaborate a little on what I call "blinders" – especially if you're feeling some resistance during this exercise. In the past, when the horse and buggy was the main mode of transportation, the horses would sometimes get distracted by activities or sudden movements to their sides, especially if a small animal jumped out of the bushes on either side of the road, as often happened. This would frighten or "spook" the horse, causing it to stop and rear up on its back legs. Buggies were sometimes overturned, or the horse would run away panicked. We've all seen the western movies with out-of-control horses pulling a carriage, the damsel in distress leaning out of the window and screaming, and the cowboy riding in to save the day, stopping the carriage just before it plummets off a cliff. But there wasn't always a hero around, so to prevent this, they began to put blinders on the horses, which removed these distractions, allowing horses to focus only on the path ahead.

Similarly, we humans have mental blinders, built over time to stay within the confines of how we were raised, programmed, and conditioned. Genetics also play a part in shaping who we think we're supposed to be.

If you were to take your finger and put it on the side of your nose, you would be able to see your finger, but not your nose. You do have the peripheral vision to see the side of your nose, so why can't you? Because your mind is automatically making the adjustments and blocking it out. Psychological blinders are no different.

To use an extreme example, an athlete named Roger Bannister was the first runner to break the four-minute mile in 1954. Soon afterward, many other runners accomplished the same feat. This was because their blinders (self-imposed limitations) were removed by the awareness that running a mile in under four minutes was possible. The same was true when, in 1970, Soviet weightlifter Vasily Ivanovich Alekseyev became the first man to lift over 500 pounds above his head. In the years that followed, numerous weightlifters did it too. Until he showed them it was possible, the 500-pound threshold was an imaginary limit.

Likewise, as our blinders are pulled away, even a little bit, we are able to do more. When you open up possibilities, it begins to expand your current paradigm – that is, what you see as impossible and possible in your own life.

So in today's training, have an open mind and allow your blinders to be removed. Tell that part of your mind that wants to help and protect you that you will be okay, that you know what you're doing, and that it can "stand down." Soon, you will be able to achieve more (and that mental security guard can finally get more R&R time.)

Now let's start the next exercise. It's called **Standing Rising Sun.**

It is similar to the last one but with some different mental imagery.

- Breathe in while expanding the belly, then breathe out while contracting the belly. The goal is to breathe mainly in that area.

- Do the movements of the exercise The Standing Tree in the previous section.

- Again, stand with your feet shoulder-width apart and your hands on your sides.

- Slowly raise your hands while inhaling deeply like a vacuum, and try to feel it in your palms. (Inhale through your nose.)

- Allow your hands to become the breath, as if you're breathing out of your hands only. (Exhale through your mouth.)

- Let your hands float down as you breathe out, slowly falling like feathers. The goal is to focus on breathing out with your hands; as you do, you should begin to feel a sensation.

- Don't forget to breathe in deeply while you raise your hands, and breathe out slowing as you lower them.

This is a great habit to begin each morning with. Perform at least three repetitions. If you're not used to breathing a little deeper, just breathe in as deeply as you can without feeling uncomfortable.

When you are performing this exercise, it is important that you understand the differences between the two exercises. The first exercise needs to be performed three to four times a week for at least two weeks before you progress to the next one.

As you review and reflect on this lesson and your meditation, open your mind to these ideas, and hear what your mind has filtered out.

I look forward to teaching you step two.

In the next chapter, we will build upon the solid foundation I mentioned earlier. The next lesson is intertwined with the first. The more you practice each step, the better you will be prepared for the next one, and the greater your results and achievement will be.

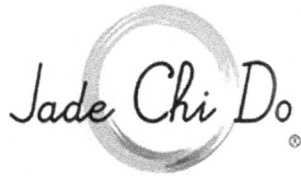

PART I - CHAPTER 2

First Steps

To those reading or listening to me - you may know who you are, but do you know *why* you are? How about *how much* you are?

In this chapter, I will discuss something I call "inner knowing". Whatever you consider your current abilities to be, they are just the tip of the iceberg. As you know, most of an iceberg is hidden below the surface of the water. This is what lies deep within you, unseen by others, and often inaccessible to you, though you can feel it pushing from below the surface of your consciousness.

To use another metaphor, imagine this inner knowing – your innate abilities, as a bird struggling to break free of an egg. It's eyes aren't even open yet. It is in total darkness. And yet somehow it yearns for the world outside of its shell. It sees the dim light and hears the mysterious murmurs, so it takes its soft beak and begins to break out. When it emerges, it doesn't take long for it to feel (even when it still doesn't "know") that it is meant for even greater things. It is meant to tuck and roll, climb and dive in the high, clear air.

What drives this instinct? Why would the vulnerable baby bird leave the safety and warmth of the egg to venture out into the unknown, outside world rather than hiding there as long as possible? Somehow, it instinctively knows that life is so much more than the dark, cramped world of the egg. It is drawn to the light.

Likewise, learning how to access your inner knowing is as natural as waking up in the morning. The next steps in your evolution are learning how, then applying what you learn consistently. It is time to flip the iceberg over. It is time to shatter your egg, burst free, and fly.

In recent years, many famous scientists have detected a quickening taking place in the world, though they have expressed it in different ways. This quantum change may have changed little in the lives of ordinary people, but it is there just the same.

Perhaps you have gone through your entire life so far knowing - or more accurately, feeling - that you are much more than what you have been able to access. You have been right. It is true. And it is time to make the extraordinary ordinary.

Though you have carried this deeper knowledge within yourself throughout your life, and you may have found ways to express yourself that were very satisfying, you may have also felt that you have not yet scratched the surface of the treasure trove that is within you. You may have even had the feeling that you're "waiting" for something to happen. Sound familiar?

There is no pressure unless something real is causing it - unless what is inside the vessel has become too large to be contained. If the pressure is not released, there will be an explosion. Or, in terms of human emotion, growing frustration, resulting in a meltdown of some kind. The only other option is to increase the size of the container.

Again, we are in a quickening, a worldwide transformation. The pressure you are feeling is building under the surface of our paradigm.

Lesson Two is a continuation of Lesson One. All the lessons in this book will overlap in this way. We'll be starting at a basic level so you may encounter confusion, but keep in mind that, again, confusion is always the doorway to higher understanding. You may also feel bored, but when this happens, remind yourself that you are building up to something amazing. As the saying goes, Rome wasn't built in a day. And you, my friend, are Rome.

Though the movements I share with you may seem simple, they are seeds that will grow into something very tangible if the soil they are planted in (your mind, heart, and soul) is fertile.

Keep your cup empty so it may be filled. If it's already full, no more can be added. This will adversely affect your results and hinder the continued outcome and potential.

Practicing these lessons frequently will increase both your untapped, innate abilities and your ability to access them. Keep your eye on the prize – finally excavating your full potential. Not part of it – all of it. You will burst in every direction like a sun. You will be a source of awe and inspiration to all who know you. And you will be forever free of that old frustration, that gnawing feeling of waiting but never arriving. You will have access to your entire self and all the gifts you were born with, as well as the gifts you have developed but lost along the way.

A student once asked, "Teacher, what is the recipe that will help me achieve that which you teach?"

The teacher responded, "It will be possible when you apply the imagination of a child, the security and discipline of an adult, and the willingness to be brave enough to let your ego rest and allow a new seed to grow from a cup that is empty. The challenge of the empty cup is that many feel naked and insecure and thus are never able to reach the fruit of accomplishment."

Let's work on our recipe.

One warm summer's day, a teacher and his student walked to the top of a hill and sat down. Looking out across the vast, green valley below, the student said, "I am baffled by the feats I have seen you perform when you're teaching. How are you able to do such things? And how do you know what is inside me? There are times when I feel like I may burst, but other times when I feel empty, barren, alone. How can I stay full? How can I find and use all that is within me? How can a seed grow out of an empty cup if it has no tea?"

The teacher looked at him, intrigued by these questions. He thought for a moment and said, "What have you been told to have - to be able to do the things you wish to do?"

The student replied, "Well, I've been told that I just need to have belief and the faith of a seed, a very small seed."

"Do you believe this?" the teacher asked.

"Well, my belief is definitely very small, so I am just like the seed. I feel I should be doing great things, but I haven't so far. What am I not seeing?"

The teacher smiled and looked at the student, "What else is a seed? If you were actually a seed and someone asked you what you are, what would you say?"

The student thought a moment and replied, "Well, a seed is what things grow from."

"Exactly!" replied the teacher. "A seed is the beginning. What does a seed do once it has water?" the teacher asked.

"It produces roots" the student answered.

"Correct," said the teacher. "It then reaches for the light in the sky and, in this case, turns into a tree. If the roots are not sound, the tree does not flourish. So what have you just learned?"

"That the success of a seed, in my case, has nothing to do with its size but the confidence in what is being taught, and its ability to grow from the new knowledge it attains."

The teacher smiled. The student asked one more question.

"Teacher, can you just give me this training ability? Why must I start out as a seed to acquire it? I want to know everything today. What must I do?"

The teacher replied, "You must be willing to start from the seed and build your confidence from there. You lose confidence when you compare yourself to others. You lose resolve and focus when you look too far into the future and become overwhelmed by the distance left to travel. Focusing completely on each step ensures success. The first step of the seed is to produce the root. The techniques I teach you will install control over your direction, which will propel you to the light at the surface."

The student sighed and said, "I suppose I am impatient, but now that I know it's possible for me to find and use everything that is within me, I am more anxious than ever."

The teacher replied, "It is better for a tree to grow at the edge of a forest. If it grows in the middle, it won't get much wind or sunlight. Never tested, its roots will be shallow and weak, not deep and wide. The first challenging wind will knock it over. Your roots are the discipline and focus you devote to your exercises. Involve your every sense completely in every moment and you will receive the full benefit of your education."

The student replied, "Teacher, I promise my cup will be empty. I will remain focused, and remind myself every day that my cup must stay empty."

The teacher smiled.

Continuation of Rising Sun.

Introduction to Sitting Rising Sun.

This Lesson is called **Sitting Rising Sun** because we do this exercise in the morning. The continuation of this lesson should be done daily. It does not have to be done only in the morning.

- Sit in a chair with your back erect and your palms on your knees.

- Lift your hands as you breathe in through your nose – again imagining breathing in through your palms – until your hands are at shoulder height.

- Slowly breathe out through your mouth and allow the air to flow out of both of your palms equally.

- Repeat this three or four times. Breathe deeply.

- Focus on the breath within your hands; that is, your entire palm and all of your fingers.

- At the end of the last set, as your hands slowly float down, just before they touch your knees, slowly turn your palms until they face each other, keeping your hands above your knees. As you do so, you will feel something. I will explain what it is shortly. For now, just continue your breathing.

- With your palms still facing each other, rest your wrist on your knees.

- Close your eyes, breathe in and out "through" your hands for a couple of breaths.

- Next, as you breathe in through your palms, expand each hand by bending a little bit outward at the wrist.

- Next, while you breathe out, push your palms slightly back in at the wrist, facing each other again. You may have a feeling of pressure between your palms. Just let it be and pay no attention to it.

- Next, continue to breathe from your palms. Doing the same exercise without moving, give yourself a slight signal to your hands, as if you're still moving each of them in and out with your breath. (It is important that there is no or minimal movement. This may sound contradictory but as we go forward, so will the depth of your understanding.) Basically, you can feel both of your palms sort of expanding outward as you're breathing, as if your hands are breathing in, like a vacuum.

- As you exhale, feel your hands and your mind compress a little bit, almost as if your hands are doing it. Compress, then breathe, then compress. You'll feel something very different between your palms. It may feel like a kind of pressure, but don't let this distract you.

Something even more wondrous is just around the corner, but the goal right now is to simply execute this exercise with full focus. Do these exercises every morning. Again, so far, they are:

1. The Standing Tree

2. Standing Rising Sun.

3. Sitting Rising sun

If you only have time for one, it is better to practice one than none at all.

Our next lesson will be **Rising Lotus,** which includes The Standing Tree, Standing Rising Sun, and Sitting Rising Sun. This is the beginning of Rising Lotus. Again, each lesson intertwines with the next. Rising Lotus has three parts.

- Start with a chair behind you to sit in later in the exercise.

- Keep your gaze forward but focus on nothing. Keep your thoughts in the moment, like a tree feeling the wind.

- Start with Standing Tree. Bend at the knees when raising your arms, and straighten your legs when moving your arms down to your sides. Inhale when raising your hands, and exhale when lowering your hands. Just normal natural breathing.

- Next, start Standing Rising Sun. That is, add the special breathing that was taught in that section.

- Next, sit on the chair behind you. Start doing Sitting Rising Sun.

- Do the previously taught breathing in the Standing Rising Sun exercise.

- Finish by standing again and repeating The Standing Tree exercise at the end of this first part of Rising Lotus. (If you are not near a chair, just exclude that part until you are near one.)

- Practice Daily until you move on to other exercises, but do practice intermittently with the others exercises you will be learning. This exercise will take on a new, greater meaning as you grow and discover more things within you.

I was teaching a student recently who asked, "Why are the exercises involving the hands and feet so important for connecting with our life force?" I believe this would be a good place to share the answer:

"We use our hands and feet to feel this world, and they transmit information to our innermost selves. The nerves in your hands sense, receive, and send information. They are always communicating, like antennae receiving and broadcasting. In basic terms, this is internal through our nerves, but we can also feel more subtle fluctuations. Jade Chi Do exercises facilitate the discovery and control of greater abilities for this receiving and broadcasting system. In other words, engaging the entire body through this training will help lower one's personal blinders so that they can find, feel, and use their innate powers in very life-transforming ways - powers that have been there all along, waiting to be discovered.

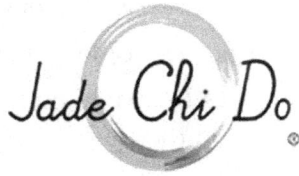

PART I - CHAPTER 3

Our Anchors

In this chapter, I will tell you about something that was brought to my attention that will help accelerate the rewards you acquire from Jade Chi Do.

I was speaking with a student one day after class and he told me he was having some challenges with focus while training. He asked me three questions:

I was speaking with a student one day after class and he told me he was having some challenges with focus while training. He asked me three questions:

1. What can I do to avoid getting distracted?

2. How do I get rid of feelings of insecurity and anxiety that are slowing the results of my training?

3. How can I heal as fast as I did when I was younger?

I was surprised by his questions. I thought for a moment and realized that the first thing I needed to do to help him get the benefits of his Jade Chi Do training was to give him some anchors. With some basic anchors in place, he would have less unconscious resistance to training and open himself up to accessing extraordinary rewards.

I also learned not to assume that a student showing up and wanting to learn means they are actually *ready* to learn.

Here are some simple but important tools I used to address the student's three questions. Let's start with attention and distractions:

In a nutshell, we need to *produce* content instead of being driven and controlled by incoming content. Distraction and loss of attention are the standard in our current environment. Our electronic world produces massive amounts of content - social media posts, TV, video games, music, email, texting, etc. – all competing for our attention. Since the advent of iPhones, the entire world literally sits in the palms of our hands. This gives an invisible yet consistent kind of pressure. If we start to do something that requires us to lead the activity instead of merely receiving it, we get tired, bored and distracted because we have become accustomed to a constant onslaught of content. As a result, most modern humans are conditioned to rely on the electronic bombardment that comes at them each day. Give most kids a book these days and they'll reject it because it doesn't light up or make noise. Sadly, that's true for most adults too.

The way to take back your mental freedom is by practicing awareness of yourself. There are simple tools (exercises) that, if given a chance, and if real effort is applied, will direct you toward freedom and control over your choices and attention. The goal is to bring awareness back to your body. Developing anchors through breathing exercises and other tools will help create foundations to branch out, empower yourself, gain control, and reach goals. However, you must first make a conscious choice to want to make a difference, and to want to achieve what lays before you - whether your daily tasks or some other endeavor.

A brick is a brick, but when you build a home, you can stack them in many different shapes and achieve many different results. Many gurus will give you a plan of action (show you how to lay a brick) but in the end, you're the one who does the work according to your own unique design. You are the only you in the whole universe, and only you know the full extent of the gifts you have within you. You may also feel that you have gifts at the surface waiting to come out, but are unsure how to access them. You will find the tools in this book to be liberating in this way and many others. They will also help you regain the control that the world has thrown out of balance. They will awaken or reawaken your ability to communicate with yourself. They will have you pushing media content away. Like anything else, it will take repetition to build strength, but the rewards will be for a lifetime and can be passed down to your loved ones. The rewards will come faster and be stronger if you approach these exercises with the ancient philosophy passed from master to master, "From the deepest sincerity comes the greatest achievement."

We start with baby steps, allowing ourselves to be more aware of what we do in every moment. Most of humanity drifts through each day, not paying attention very closely, filling their time with mostly mindless activity. These things aren't inherently bad; it's the lack of consciousness that is harmful. If we develop a relationship with and awareness of these activities, we are more empowered to steer away from a stalled and distracted lifestyle.

Reaffirming the power of choice within us is very rewarding. These short, simple tools will strengthen your life and put you back in the driver's seat; that is, fully aware of what you are doing with your time.

Do not let the simplicity of the following tools make you think they are simple or ineffective. In time, if you are patient and sincere in your practice, you will learn how truly powerful they are. Is it not this way with all things? Most people look at the Grand Canyon and see only its depth and width. They don't see the million years of wind and flowing water that carved it. So which is stronger – the stone, or the wind and water?

Let's begin:

- Get a piece of paper or a notebook, and a pencil or pen.

- Draw six circles big enough for you to write a sentence in.

- Above the circles, write a time in the morning and a time in the evening when you know you'll have 30 seconds for this exercise. Three of the circles will contain morning questions; the other three will contain evening questions.

- Write in the first "morning" circle, "The immediate goals I want to get done today."

- On the evening side, write, "Did I accomplish these goals today?"

- In the next morning circle, write, "I will meditate today."

- In the next evening question, write, "Did I make time to meditate today?"

- In the last morning circle, write, "I am going to exercise today."

- In the next evening circle, write, "Did I exercise today?"

- Each day, on the next page, write the current date, "Yes" or "No", and the goals you want to obtain.

- Do this for two weeks. If you find it's working for you, continue it for the next thirty days.

- At the end of each week, add up all the yes answers and compare it to the number of times you answered no. Give it a percentage. Your goal is to keep improving week by week until you have nothing but "yes" on your list. I am confident you will find this to be a very empowering and liberating tool.

The next thing my student asked about was anxiety. There's a secret that gurus and large companies with cookie-cutter meditations don't tell you – that anxiety is unique to the individual. There's no one certain thing that will erase anxiety for everyone. What triggers and alleviates anxiety is different from one person to another. I don't know what your anxiety triggers are, nor what may be the best avenue to alleviate them, but here's a tailored plan for you.

This exercise is called **Calming Waves.**

- Choose a moment when you are not in extreme anxiety.

- Find a picture that moves you and look at that picture every day.

- Take a deep breath and hold it for a second or two.

- Exhale as you look at the picture while it gives you that good feeling.

- Stop looking at that picture, but remember the feeling.

- If the feeling goes away, look at the picture again and remind yourself. Feel the good emotions again like a ray of sunshine shining on you. Feel the warmth and good feelings deeply.

- Turn the picture over (or your phone, if that's where it is.) Visualize the photo and try to feel the emotion it evokes again. This is the purpose of this exercise - recalling the memory of that good feeling.

- Next, choose a picture that does NOT make you feel sad, such as a loved one who has passed away; one that moves you and communicates something deep within you. For some people, that might be a beautiful sunset. For you, it may be a field of wildflowers, or a majestic mountain. Whatever it is, it should feel unique to you and trigger a feeling of awe, of coming home, of warmth, but again, no sadness, loneliness, or missing somebody.

- Do this exercise five or six times a day, every day.

A student once showed me her special photo. It was a bunch of pumpkins that were all the colors of autumn. For some reason known only to her, that connected with her on a deep emotional level and made her feel positive, warm, and happy. She was able to gain control over many painful emotions with this exercise. She would look at the picture, feel the warm emotion connected with it, then turn the picture over (or close her eyes) and remember the feeling. She preferred closing her eyes, but I suggested turning the picture over and working on remembering the feeling with her eyes open too. **When you do this exercise, you are building a tool you will be able to use for a lifetime.**

Important: Do not stare at the picture too long at one time. The purpose of the exercise is not to memorize the photo as much as it is to carry or stretch out the memory of the emotion it elicits. Look at the photo for a very short moment, then work on the emotional memory of it. You will find that your ability to do this will become increasingly stronger with repetition, and because of your will (choice).

It is best to practice this when you're not anxious, but you can also use it to calm yourself when you are. Remember, all things have opposites. Happy and sad, dark and bright, etc. Likewise, just as you have an anxiety trigger, you also have a calming trigger. We are going to take control of this and build your trigger. You can use this at the moment you feel your anxiety trigger being pulled. Remember, in this world of opposites, if it can go one way for you, you must know in your heart that it can just as easily go the other way. With this exercise, you're going to reinforce that feeling.

The moment your anxiety starts, take a deep breath, and as you exhale, see/feel your picture and let the warm, happy feeling it gives you fill you up, as if you were very thirsty and you just had a drink of cold water. You will find that this quick little secret works extremely well. There are other things you can do to deal with anxiety, but like the lady who shared her photo of fall pumpkins with me, this one exercise was so powerful, it changed her life forever.

I hope you'll accept this secret, from my heart to yours. I look forward to helping you become the explorer that you are, and to reminding you that there's more. You will no longer have to sit and watch the world go by, like a party you weren't invited to. It is time for you to become very active with the world, starting within yourself. This secret is an anchor for you, just like a boat's anchor, preventing the waves (emotions) from turning you over and carrying you causing you to crash on the rocks (anxiety). Now that you have an anchor, I invite you to work on the boat that will help you navigate through the sea of life.

The third and last comment my student gave me was that he didn't heal as fast as he thought he should, or as fast as he did when he was young.

When we're young, small cuts heal in about seven days, and colds don't usually last more than a few days. As we get older, we tend to take longer to heal or feel better. However, the reason for this is not always only age but lifestyle as well.

Here is a starting point that has helped me a lot with this. The moment your skin is cut, your body is notified and healing starts. We are immediately notified about the pain. So, the key at this stage is attention. To use another example, when we hear a car alarm going off, the noise travels to our ears, which gets our **Attention.** At that point, we can take **Action** by either distancing ourselves from the alarm so that we don't hear it anymore, or going toward it to shut it off. Likewise, we can fix or pull a tooth, but either way, it needs to heal. It will be sore for some time. Therefore, the third stage is **Time**. To heal faster, we must combine these three ingredients – action, attention, and time.

In regard to wounds that can heal naturally, like cuts and other injuries, we must shorten the time needed by maintaining our attention to it. Here is another simple exercise that will start to give you this ability. I call it **Applying the Three Ingredients - Attention, Action, and Time.**

- Sit in a comfortable chair and recognize the spot where the hurt is. For this example, we're using a cut.

- Maintain your attention with the breath of attention. Connect your breath to whatever it is that is causing you pain. Breathe in as if you're inhaling into the hurt, then exhale as if you're blowing out the hurt. Facing the hurt instead of running from it will continue to keep the attention upon it. This helps the body keep an open awareness of its duties to naturally heal. This has an effect on the last ingredient.

The more often you practice this exercise, the faster your healing process will be. This is a strong but simple exercise that is very rewarding when actively practiced. Its benefits are accelerated and expanded by in-depth training in the practice of Jade Chi Do.

These three questions from my student highlighted to me the importance of getting one's whole life in order so we can understand

and build upon what we learn. We will continue toward this goal in the following chapters.

Our next chapter will start our moving meditations. Why include motion in meditation? *A live cell is always moving. Life does not stand still.* Therefore, adding internal and external motion to your static meditations is highly recommended. This increases health and awareness. The training contained here will open up a higher awareness of yourself and the life force within you.

You May Be Wondering . . . Why Practice Flowing Movements?

Flowing movements achieve two things on the bio-electrical side of the body. They maintain a continual current, reinforcing the nervous system, which is good at any age. They also build a greater response time in sports and speed up recovery time when accidents occur. A constant field of flowing energy also removes tension from the body. Freedom of motion is the opposite of tension. Even in combat, movements that flow like a ball rolling will connect the trained techniques and control the challenge in most cases. Many times, the opponent will impose his counterattack in the break of your flow. But beyond combat, a flowing bio-electrical system is crucial to one's health.

Clumsy movements in regular life are often described as "stop-and-go". Take the example of picking up a cup. I look at the cup and give myself a command of sorts to reach for it and pick it up. Sometimes my mind jumps ahead to what I am going to do next, causing me to lose focus on what I'm doing at that moment. By doing this, I may bump another cup or even tip it over. By practicing full attention to this, after some time, one can reset this ability to become automatic and more graceful. Test it! You will see for yourself.

Jade Chi Do

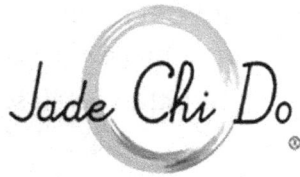

PART I - CHAPTER 4

Heaven And Earth

I n this session, we will explore the metaphor of the tree, and go a little bit further into it. Trees have long been used as symbols for virtuous traits and causes. Poems have been written about them. Many think of a tree as a great symbol for life – firmly rooted and strong, but always reaching out. Whether you have similar thoughts or your own unique views about trees, for the purpose of this training, we're using the tree as a symbol of the person within you.

What are the first things we notice about a tree? Generally, it grows upward toward the sun. It stays aligned with gravity. The roots go deep into the earth, giving the tree above stability while staying connected to the earth, from which it draws its nourishment. As the tree reaches upward, its branches reach out, and its leaves reach out even further. The leaves are like a million little solar panels, soaking up energy from the sun. A tree begins to grow upward as soon as it sprouts out of the seed, but what tells the tree which direction is up? Yes, the sun, but because it can't see the sun when planted deep underground, it is guided even more by gravity, our earth's natural energy. The sprout never emerges from the earth at an angle. A tree always seeks alignment.

As you may have heard, having good posture is very important, but aligning with gravity and connecting with the earth is too. This new exercise – **Heaven and Earth** - is the first moving exercise. It connects and aligns us. Creating this sensitivity is very important. You will notice that once you are well rooted with heaven and earth, you can feel the motion when you walk. The benefits are highly cumulative and very rewarding. When you reach a certain point, you will want to do this every day. Now, on to our meditation.

Moving Exercise #1 - Heaven and Earth.

This exercise will be divided into three sections:

1. Lower: performed just above the height of your hips.

2. Middle: performed around shoulder height.

3. Upper: performed overhead.

- Stand with your feet shoulder-width apart, your head and shoulders as erect as possible, knees slightly bent, hands on your side, palms facing your hips and your fingers pointing down.

- Deeply relax your hands and arms.

Next, you will begin to use your breath exercise, and this will form the beginning training exercises.

Lower:

- Connect your breath, and as you breathe in, allow your arms to go out like wings with a slow, smooth motion but no more than approximately 1½ feet outward, or about halfway between having your arms straight out to each side and level with the floor.

- Keep your palms facing inward.

- Breathe in as your arms move away from your body. Feel the energy coming in, as if you're breathing in through your hands. (Your whole focus is on the reality of feeling, imagining, and visualizing only this, with no other thoughts. You should be sensitive to this feeling now from practicing earlier lessons. If not, go back and build your foundation stronger to connect more powerfully to this.)

- As you breathe out, bring your hands in toward your legs. Do not touch your legs. As you bring your hands in, feel and visualize breathing or "pushing" the energy out through your hands.

As you go further in your training, you will feel a growing and very different sensation in your palms and the bottom of your feet as energy differentiates itself from your breath. Over time, with each new exercise and form you learn, this will intensify and become very strong and useful. This frequency vibration I share with you will not be hidden anymore. This force will have its own feeling. It will no longer be connected just to your breath.

To return to this exercise:

- As your arms lower, consciously push and feel your breath moving through your feet. As you do this and your arms go in, feel the energy of your breath pushing out. As you push your hands in, you'll feel and see the direction of your mind going out of your feet. You will feel a sort of pressure.

- Take a soft breath as you breathe out. You will feel like there's something between your hands and legs. As your hands collapse down, you'll feel it going through your feet into the earth. Like a tree, you are now rooting, standing erect, and aligning with gravity.

- Now breathe in and expand your arms and hands like wings opening, as if it's the wind pushing in.

- At the same time, inhale with your palms and feet.

- Next, lower your hands, slightly pushing your breath out of your hands and feet, rooting into the earth as your hands drop, again like wings. Feel the pressure and all the energy as you breathe out, pushing your breath out of your hands and through your feet. With practice, this rooting part will feel natural.

Repeat this exercise three times.

Now we're going to do it again, but with breathing that is a little different.

- Breathe in through your nose, inhaling into your belly. (Fill your lower abdomen first, but fill your lungs more deeply as you get better at this exercise.) Remember, you're exhaling out of your hands and feet - one or both - depending on the exercise.

- Breathe out of your mouth as you lower your arms. (Always pushing.)

- When you breathe in through your nose, keep your tongue on the roof of your mouth to shut off mouth breathing.

- Now, lower your tongue and breathe out of your mouth. As you do so, visualize that you're compressing your breath energy as you go down. You will then feel and visualize the breath energy going out of your hands and feet, giving direction of movement to your whole body. If done correctly, the more you practice this, the stronger you will feel.

Practice this a few times so you get the feeling. When you do the Heaven and Earth exercise, you can do this one beginning exercise without using your legs as a builder. I call this rooting. I use this a lot before exercises to align and empower because it creates a trigger for a strong zone for great achievement. Again, visualize your rooting as tree roots going down into the earth, securing the tree above.

Let's move on to the next step. Start by doing the rooting exercise three times, then the regular Heaven and Earth exercise. You can root any time just by doing the building exercise and rooting.

- When you raise your hands up like wings, sink a little, bending at the knees. You can judge how low or high you go depending on your health, strength, flexibility, etc. This will increase with time and practice. In the future, you will be able to bend a lot further and do the same breathing, but for now, just do a gentle bend.

- As your hands rise up, bend down to receive energy from the earth just like the roots of a tree suck up nutrients. Likewise, your feet, palms, and the earth inhale the energy of life around us.

- Feel your breath go into your hands and up through your feet.

- Lower your hands back down, like gentle wings floating downward, flowing, growing, and rooting. At the same time, all the energy is pushing through your feet as you stand back up.

- As your hands rise up, your knees bend, then come back down and stand up. Let your knees get close to locking out, but not all the way.

- As you drop your hands, push just like you're pushing energy into the earth - pushing energy from your hands out, going down. This is just like the rooting exercise except you're using your knees as well.

To recap:

- Stand with your legs shoulder-width apart.

- Do the rooting exercise with your hands on your sides, palms facing your hips.

- Slowly raise your relaxed hands as you breathe in. Feel the energy in your hands.

- Lower your hands as you breathe out. Feel the energy of your breath coming out of your hands, going down your legs, and out of your feet as well.

- Do this exercise three times.

- Open your eyes and gaze straight ahead.

You can also do this with your eyes closed if your balance is good. If you did the entire exercise with your eyes closed, do it again in whole or in part with your eyes open to increase balance and other benefits.

Just as the tree gathering nutrients through its roots is part of its energy, so too do we gather energy from the earth. During each part of the exercise, visualize seeing your breath as energy blowing outward from your hands and feet. Breathe in through your nose and out through your mouth. Your body should be calm. Monitor your body for any tension. Don't fight it; allow it to relieve itself as you let it go, and send it away through your breath.

Middle section

- Flowing from the "lower part" exercise, raise your hands upward from your sides. For this entire exercise, keep your hands and arms on your sides, not to the front or back.

- As you inhale, raise your hands and bend your knees, but this time, raise your hands all the way to shoulder height.

- Slightly bend your knees while inhaling, then inhale just a little more and pull your hands back with your palms away from your head.

- Now that your hands are close to your shoulders, push out like you're pushing two walls, with your palms facing outward, fingers close together, pointing up. (The pushing is as if you're standing in a doorway with both palms actually pushing outward on the door frame.)

- While pushing out, breathe out as you stand up from your knees, which are still bent from the prior inhale.

- Visualize your breath going out of your hands and feet into the earth, your surroundings, and infinity.

- Do it again.

- Drop to the elbows.

- Keep your palms facing outward, relaxed.

- Breathe out.

Upper - overhead (still flowing)

- Next, as you are moving your arms outward from your sides, raise your hands up until they're right above your head. Your palms should be facing up and your fingertips facing each other just above your head.

- At the same time, breathe in and sink with your knees on the inhale.

- As you breathe out, push up with your palms up, like you're holding a pizza pan.

- At the same time, straighten your legs, pushing your breath energy out of your feet down into the earth.

Have you figured out - or more accurately, felt - what's happening as you do this exercise? You are creating opposing energy - your hands to heaven and your feet to earth – with the use of opposing directions of breath. Breath is really just energy. When you visualize the flow, you increase this energy. This is Heaven and Earth.

You should have the feeling that you're pushing your breath out through your feet as you raise your hands up until both fingers are pointing toward each other. When your palms are pointing to heaven, breathe out. (Again, your hands are flat, like you're holding a pizza pan.) You are sending your breath energy out of your hands to heaven and down to earth at the same time. Visualize and feel this.

- When you have done this three times, slowly let your arms down, with your hands and fingers pointing toward each other.
- Breathe in.
- Slightly bend your knees.
- Continue to lower your arms with your elbows leading, first down to your sides, then your hands follow, palms outward.
- Push out - again, like pushing outward inside a door frame.

Do this middle exercise three times.

- At the end of the final push, let your hands fall like falling wings to the first lower rooting exercise position.

The object is to do each of these three sections three times each. Start by doing the rooting exercise, then the middle exercise, then the overhead exercise, three times each. Then do it in reverse: The overheard, middle, and rooting exercise, again three times each.

- Do the rooting exercise three times with slightly bent knees, then just the rooting with knees not locked and not moving.

- When you're done, let your hands fall to your sides gently, like wings floating down. Practice very slowly, feeding each motion, connected to your breathing, with energy and direction coming from your palms and feet.

That is the exercise. Once you begin to really follow the movements and engage all your senses, you will feel like you're in a zone of extreme focus. The benefits are very rewarding and you will start to feel them right away, or within a few days. Many of my students have been surprised and even afraid of the power they felt as a result of this exercise. But there's nothing to be afraid of. It's just your body and mind doing what they were always capable of. These abilities just needed to be unlocked.

I invite you to review my site for further information. You can find training videos on this which may be very helpful. Please also check the accompanying illustrations there.

Main goals
- Pay attention to every moment, every motion, and your breathing.

- Feel your hands and feet with your breath.

- Make each movement very smooth, with no interruption. When transitioning into any movement, the goal should be no hesitation or stop-and-go, jerky motions. However, don't be hard on yourself if there are. We never really reach the point where there's absolutely no breakage, but our goal is to continually strive for that.

If your balance is good, do this exercise at first with your eyes closed. This will help you align with the force of gravity and all of the energies and the electrical system within your body. After doing this for some time, it will feel like flicking a light switch to the on position. It is incredibly empowering when you feel the alignment happen. When you are "in the moment" in this exercise, it will feel as if time has no meaning; a zone like no other.

- After you do the exercise with closed eyes, your goal is to continue the rooting. (The beginning of the exercise). If time permits, do the exercise with your eyes open and feel focused. You will notice something interesting and exciting - a greater sense of control.

- To finish, at the very end, when you're doing the rooting exercise again, open your eyes and just root, gazing straight ahead.

Try to feel these feelings and your attention to them with your eyes open. The better you get, the easier it will be to do both. But again, if your balance is a little off when you close your eyes, continue to practice with your eyes open and just visualize it. Maintaining focus - what your attention is on - is very important. In the end, your attention will be on all of it at once, as if you're gazing at something without your eyes focused on one thing but viewing the picture as a whole.

The best time to practice this is anytime that feels good to you, but I have found the greatest success and acceleration in the early morning just after I wake. You can do this exercise in the dark, with your eyes closed, or with your eyes slightly open.

This exercise will help you achieve greater benefits and amplify the "zone" effect, which will then extend into all your activities. Being able to get into a special zone to achieve one's goals is phenomenal whether you apply this to sports, gaming, entrepreneurship, or life in general.

I recommend also doing this exercise in water. A swimming pool is best for water stillness and temperature control. With the water up to your neck, do the exercise in slow motion. This will help your balance and show you where your motion is breaking instead of flowing. The goal is always smooth, flowing motion. Doing the grounding exercises of Heaven and Earth in the shower will also help. It should be done very slowly, with a clear mind; no thought, just observing everything visually but not focused on anything. Then, breathe in through your hands as they come out like wings just a foot away from your hips, your palms and fingers pointing down and palms facing the body. In extremely slow motion, inhale through your hands and go back in and toward your hips. Feel the lifeforce going out to your hands and down your legs to the earth. When done in this zone, you will feel your hands ignite, as well as a magnetic sensation.

Adding water to this exercise is very rewarding, especially when you have begun to recognize the warm force and internally define it. You will also notice that your training will rapidly improve afterward.

Another important way to accelerate your progress is through diet and exercise. When I use the term diet, I don't mean eating more or less; I mean the foods you eat. We have all heard that our body has to process everything we eat. I have found that a diet high in alkaline and healthy oils like organic liquid coconut oil amplifies your training. Please do your own research on the above diet. When following this diet, your body will respond well to exercise and the training in this book. The results will speak for themselves.

Additional training note:

We have a special VR app for training! Go here to get into our beta testing group, or visit: www..JadeChiDo.app

VR has its place, but one must train this in the "RW" (Real World) as well to physically interact with the current, perceived world around us. The VR experience can compliment Jade Chi Do in opening the door to more and greater discoveries, but it is crucial to do the exercises (again, in the RW) to expand what we see within our current physical world.

Jade Chi Do

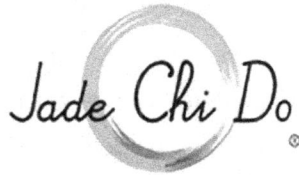

PART I - CHAPTER 5

The Champion's Zone

Secret Tool

What if I told you that you could be in the zone, exactly as many athletes claim to be when they're performing at their highest level, and that it will become a common daily experience for you to know the pure fulfillment of a successfully completed action?

The zone time has no meaning. Your self listens to you all the time. The combination of your words, actions, and thoughts combine to translate into a special language that speaks to the inner, serving self. To use a previous example, it waits while you sleep to wake you up five minutes before the alarm clock. The same is true of more complex actions. This special, inner, serving self has its own language, a pure variation of infinite and complex combinations of frequencies which come from you and your choices, knowingly or unknowingly. Therefore, the words we speak and connect with emotionally communicate much.

How does this apply to Jade Chi Do? This is one of the keys for creating a clear channel of communication with yourself. This zone creates the right environment to complete a calibration to achieve maximum results. The good news is, getting into this zone is not only for gurus or famous sports stars. Anyone can do it, if they know how. When you're done reading this book, you will.

We'll start this lesson on a clear path so it won't take years to attain mastery as it once did. Your path will be much shorter and faster. There are three requirements:

1. Dedicated practice with the open mind of a child.

2. Applied repetition.

3. Daily exercise at roughly the same time.

We prioritize our listening. Have you ever caught yourself not listening to a loved one or friend in conversation? They may have said "Did you hear me?" after asking you a question you didn't hear or respond to. You probably then answered, "Could you repeat that?"

Sound familiar? I'm not referring to being tired, hearing impairment, or even having a short attention span. Obviously, you didn't hear their question because your attention was elsewhere. Your thoughts were louder than the real sounds coming from the person you were with. Even though that person is very important to you, through your emotions, you somehow gave priority to something else. When this happened, your inner self was working on something else for you. This happens because your inner self prioritizes your attention to help you achieve what you feel is important. Therefore, missing parts of what a loved one is saying doesn't mean you don't care about them; prioritizing is just what your serving self does.

This exercise is a simple but very important tool. In a short time, one can be in the zone of great athletes, artists, and entrepreneurs who use this tool every day. Some use it without even knowing it. If this is you, your ability is about to be amplified. I am going to teach you some basics to ease you into some training exercises.

Have you ever had a conversation with someone that was so interesting and exhilarating that the hours seemed to fly by and felt like no time at all? The properties of time are affected by our perception of it. We've all heard the old expression "A watched kettle never boils." Or, as Albert Einstein put it, "When you sit with a nice girl for two hours, you think it's only a minute, but when you sit on a hot stove for a minute, you think it's two hours." He was referring to relativity, but it applies equally well to time.

In the morning, I fill my coffee pot with water from my refrigerator. The water is filtered so it takes longer to fill the pitcher than it would if I used the faucet. If I watch it fill and I have a task I'm anxious to get started on, it seems to take forever. But if I read a newspaper clipping on the fridge and forget to watch the water, it seems to fill so fast, it sometimes nearly overflows.

If we were told that a great deal of money would be sent to us in a year, to most it would feel like that year was taking forever to pass. On the other hand, if we knew some horrible event was going to happen to us in a year, to most it would feel like that year was going by too fast.

What I'm about to teach you is not new. However, as I mentioned in the previous chapter, though two buildings can be made of the same kind of bricks, how they are laid determines the appearance of what is created. So, follow me in this slightly different construction and you will achieve wondrous results, the same kind of results achieved by millionaires in all walks of life. These people often talk about a strange and powerful zone that comes over them, so their ability to secure that result and perform at the highest level really just depends on their ability to enter the zone.

Here's the tool. In this exercise, you must understand each step to practice it well. If you do, your particular zone will become your greatest conduit toward a successful life in all that you do. These secret tools will propel you quickly to the zone of champions.

Secret Tool #1: Zone Exercises

Remember, though the bricks are the same, how we stack them determines their collective look, strength, and effect. It is my job to teach you the philosophy and practice of Jade Chi Do and show you the exercises that can release all of its richest benefits. It is your job to make the choice to commit and take action. Be sure to maintain an empty cup. Again, do not let the apparent simplicity of these exercises fool you. They are the doorway to extraordinary powers that you're about to tap into.

The Beginning: Building an Anchor and Root

Zone Exercise 1

This first exercise will be your trigger.

- Sit in a chair, preferably with arms you can rest your elbows and forearms on. If you don't have a chair like this, a regular chair will do. (If so, rest them on the top of your legs with your wrist past the end of your knees, palms facing the floor or ground.)

- While sitting, rest your elbows and forearms and keep your palms facing down on the arms of the chair.

- Slide your arms forward far enough for your palms to be away from the end of the rails while still facing the floor.

- For now, just look at one of your hands. (Right or left; later it can be both. You may find at times that you only have access to one hand due to work, sports, etc. This exercise can be a quick sync to oneself.)

- Start to breathe in and out of your hands in slow motion.

- When you inhale, lift your palms at the wrist.

- Lower your palms during the exhale until they are motionless and parallel with the floor.

- Breathe only through your nose.

Here is the key that builds the trigger.

- To bring attention to the movements, look at your hand or hands. Next, while doing the exercise, slow the movement. (A slow flowing motion).

- Take still, slow breaths. Be sure to maintain your visualizations. You may feel something in your palms. Do not give attention to that; just allow it to exist. Inhale a fraction of a second quicker as the palms rise to almost facing away like a wave, but not to a tight, stiff ending. Stop and reverse direction before this happens, creating a smooth, flowing transition.

- While strongly inhaling, again imagine your breath is a vacuum, inhaling energy from your hands. (Later, you can add your feet periodically.)

- On the slow inhale section, start raising your toes and front of your foot with your heel still on the ground. Lower on the exhale the same as your heels. Be sure to start the exercise just with your hands. At this time, the feet are optional.

Note: In a number of other exercises, you breathe out of your mouth, but in this special, condensing exercise, you do not. Its first purpose is to be a trigger to open up. Think of it this way: When turning on their training before combat, a soldier would gather energy but not give any signals to the opposition of his movement, breathing in with the belly only, with no sign of weakness.

A little background, and a secret:

This exercise will show you how some triumphant warriors could quickly condense and gather not only their outward skills but those which they had trained within them. A trained warrior could strike with a sword in a fraction of the time it would take for his opponent to defend himself. The best moment to utilize this speed was when he would see his opponent's chest rise as he was breathing in.

As every fighter knows, a fight is usually won or lost in that space - that moment where one "gets the jump" on the other. If one strikes you on an inhale, it takes more time to react and unify the energy going out. (This can be changed through proper training.) To hide this and be prepared requires breathing with the nose and just the belly, without raising the chest.

Try to inhale while punching a bag. You'll see what I'm talking about. Another reason someone should not strike on the inhale is that it puts the body in an unprepared state and takes more time to react, especially without proper training. I talk about this in terms of combat but this also works for sports, business, gaming, life, etc. To excel in any area, one must first understand this. Follow with an empty cup (mind) and you will go further than you have ever imagined.

A student said to me one day, "I haven't been able to achieve the great and amazing feats you speak of, but I am excelling now."

I asked the student, "What changed?"

He said, "You were teaching me, but at first, most of what I heard was my ego doing the translating as if what you were teaching was a foreign language. It was like a filter, so I was not truly interpreting all that was being taught. As I think back, all I was doing was comparing this to what I thought it was, or what I already knew. I would sometimes smugly say to myself *I've heard this before* because it was similar to something else I had learned. But later, I would discover that I was not understanding the process, or seeing the whole picture, because I was distracted by the individual ingredients. In many cases, they weren't even what I was thinking, and I would think, *How did I not see that message/lesson? I would be so much further ahead.*"

When the student shared this with me, I told him I was happy he was making progress and told him, as I would tell you, "If you happen to be the one who learns this, share it with others to help them accelerate and grow to new heights.

Okay, back to the exercise.

The best time to do this exercise is in the early morning because the most natural and quiet time is when you first wake up, but any quiet time will do. Again, it can be done at any moment of the day, or before a required action. Time may seem to drag at first, but the more you do this exercise and the better you get at it, thirty minutes will fly by and feel like five minutes. Practice it for a few minutes to build a trigger. Remember to use only nose breathing.

(Please note: Due to the perfection of triggers, doing the exercise even momentarily will create a very strong effect.) After your practice time, you will be able to do this zone exercise anytime, anywhere, while doing any activity; for instance, while holding a coffee cup with both hands and sitting in a chair. Zone exercises will accelerate your progress with Jade Chi Do, moving toward massive results in a shorter time.

Zone Exercise 2

- Sit in a comfortable chair with both hands open and facing up, resting on your thighs or a table.

- Close your eyes and breathe in.

- While breathing out, close your fingers very slowly, timed with your breath, without touching your palms.

- As you breathe in, open your hands in slow motion, repeating the same timing with your breath, breathing out and in through your palms. Feel this. Reference earlier exercises if necessary.

This also has the ability to slow and calm the body, even to the point of slowing your heartbeat. The more you practice the art, the more the door to your training opens. This exercise is a quick trigger. Once you start getting into the zone, you will know and feel it. Thereafter, you can use one hand to catch and calm any anxiety, and much more.

The next exercise will make this ability much stronger and help you use it in all facets of your life.

Zone Exercise 3

These exercises should be done together. I just choose to teach them separately because it will accelerate your results to get the movements and breath connection memorized well at first.

- Close your eyes but follow the instructions step by step until you get this down in your mind.

- Visualize: For a minute or so, imagine you're a radio. You are the music playing your favorite song. What would you do if another sound outside of your radio was a little too loud, and you could not turn that sound down or off? Would you turn up your radio a little bit to be louder than the competing sound? Most would say yes.

Note: Do not be tempted to race ahead of me; the best way to get the best results is to follow all the exercises as written.

Now you're going to turn the volume up by building a trigger. A simple secret when you start to do these exercises is to do them intensely throughout. Visualize and physically execute them, applying a slow-motion effect. Put all your attention on the exercises. If you do them correctly, with intense attention, this will be communicated to your inner self, and it will back you up - Big Time - so much so that the zone will continue to pop out of you and start showing itself in everything you do, not just sports or business. You will see it in many things. This zone is powerful. With further practice, you will see its by-product become a powerful tool you can easily access and use in all areas of your life.

A key to accelerate your progress:

Practicing a combination of the properly-executed exercises I teach you will amplify and accelerate the effects. The results will be surprising and very fulfilling. Wondrous gifts will show themselves within you.

Question: What if everything I am teaching you here has the potential to get results x10? What would you do? You will only know if you do these exercises consistently and intensely. Keeping your cup empty at all times will ensure the greatest results in the shortest amount of time.

It is too easy for us to relate to what we know and not even hear or read anything else.

This does help at times, but not when learning. The best way to get the best and fastest results is to maintain an open mind - receptive, not gullible - adventurous, not trapped within the walls of one's own understanding. The wisest man is not the one who knows everything (which is impossible), he is the one who knows there is always more to learn. If you have read this far and performed your exercises with sincerity, you know it is time!

The next chapter will expand your communication with your inner self. It will put it on your side and reduce confusion. If the upcoming information feels too stuffy and makes you feel like you're not ready to work on this now, hang in there! There's a great story coming afterward. It is said that one can hear one voice in a room full of voices, if you have your inner self on board. Let's move forward. Are you ready?

Jade Chi Do

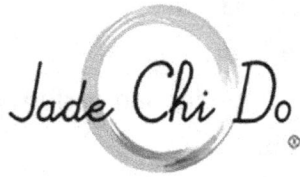

PART I - CHAPTER 6

The Art Of Awareness: To Grab The Falling Cup

Y our best communication with your inner serving self is to create a smooth pathway to developing awareness in the direction of something greater within yourself, which you may feel is already there waiting for you.

This section will create a better connection and accelerate progress for those who are serious. I will present exercises that seem simple but that may trigger certain events when practicing previous chapters at the same time.

This is where the journey starts:

The Awakening

What if you could have the full complement of focus, awareness, and intuition that your profession, sport, or martial arts style demands?

The most important thing that distinguishes one knife from others is its blade. In human terms, your blade is your focused attention and intention. Some people call it an "edge over the competition". Each style/profession is polished by the guidance you follow or have followed, whether from tradition or your interpretation. But even if you have achieved the grandest heights of your style/profession, haven't you always felt, and still feel - or somehow know - that there is more yet to be drawn from the knowledge you have mastered? Do you not feel that there is always more to learn, and that maybe this lost or as yet unattainable knowledge has eluded you in a time of need? I write this for you and anyone else who knows that there is "something else" beyond that which is knowable – a power within that you have not been able to fully access.

This book is written to be climbed like a ladder or staircase. Each chapter is designed to give you the proper insight to gradually unlock that which is within you. Thus, no chapter can be skipped or the results will be incomplete and not as rewarding.

I also write this with the goal of making these concepts tangible to you. If they are not, it is an indication that you were not "reading in the moment" – you were racing ahead, or thinking of something else. If this occurs, return to the beginning of the ladder (book) and read it again with a clear, empty, totally present mind. Your reward at the end of the book will be equivalent to the degree of your commitment; that is, the degree to which you do not let the volume of your thoughts be greater than what you are reading. The same is true in conversation - if you race ahead of someone speaking to you, there's a good chance you will also miss the point or message of what they're saying.

There is some instruction here but a great story to follow.

To See the Falling Cup

In this section, we will discuss the difference between the self and you, between intention and attention. What you *think* is not as important as what your attention is on, especially when it comes to the self. The self is a part of us that is there to serve our needs. We tend to confuse it with who we are. An example of the self at work is the internal alarm clock I mentioned before, when you tell yourself you need to wake up at a certain time and set your alarm, only to wake up just minutes or seconds before the alarm was set to ring. You were not awake to watch the clock all night, but your *self* was. Or maybe you forgot someone's name during a conversation and gave up all hope of remembering it, but then the name popped into your mind when you weren't even thinking about it. These are just hints at the unlimited power your self possesses.

If you have the power to keep track of time down to the minute, what else can you do? This is just the outer fringe, the slightest suggestion of the self that is there to serve you. My goal is to increase your communication with this source and help unlock your own personal gifts and abilities. You are greater than you are now. Now is the time to awaken the vast treasure trove that is within you, and always has been.

In life, we tend to think ahead of the moment to prepare ourselves for what's next; but by doing that, we miss or at least slow our reaction to what is really happening right in front of us. What are we telling the

Self? Have you ever read something and had to read it again because your thoughts of yesterday, tomorrow, or even today were too loud?

Let's look at this in terms of martial arts. Have you ever watched a fight and felt that one fighter "psyched out" the other one, meaning he messed with his mind so much that his attention was not in the moment? Staying in the moment is important in all things - it is just more obvious (and dangerous) in the octagon to let one's mind become distracted, whether by self-doubt or something else. I am not saying don't plan ahead, but when the moment arrives, you must be grounded and completely there. It's like studying a map to know where you're going, but then closing your eyes as you drive. Something bad is going to happen.

If the self is there to help you with your needs, then your intention and attention must be clear to it. There will be many exercises in this book, with some slight differences. They are intentional and purposeful. Practice what is similar and what is different.

A few recommendations:

- Again, drop what you think you know or have read about intention and attention so that you can install the principles of this book without interference or self-sabotage.

- Keep an open perspective about what you are reading. Try not to relate what you already know to it. Just enjoy where these simple steps can really take you.

- Keep a daily journal of your thoughts in response to the exercises in this book, or anything else that you feel is significant.

- If it fits you better, read the book first, then read it a second time while keeping a journal. It will greatly amplify your results. It not only gives you a record, it gives you a way to measure your improvement. It is also proof of your progress, which is important because it's easy to forget where you started when your abilities become greater.

You will notice that some exercises are very simple. Keep in mind that you are working in a special order and format, with your attention and intention, to help open up a bridge of clear communication with yourself.

PLEASE NOTE:

These exercises are shared as an additional resource to expand your perception. They are separate from our Jade Chi Do moving exercises. I do specify to exercise once or twice a day; however, I know you may have a busy life so if necessary, spread out the following exercises and fit them in as best you can. They will accelerate the results and quality of your Jade Chi Do moving exercises. Again, there will be a teaching story after this section to help illustrate these concepts.

Exercise 1: The Cornerstone (AKA The Blank Paper)
Step one:

- Sit at a table.

- Have nothing on the table but a blank, white piece of paper. Use a regular 8½" x 11" sheet. (Or whatever you have. It can be smaller or larger.)

Step two:

- Put the paper right in front of you and look at it.

- Say to yourself, "The paper is blank because I choose it to be."

- Continue to say only "the paper is blank" out loud as you look at the paper. Other thoughts will try to enter your mind, like what you're doing later or what is on TV. Ignore anything that may stop you from just saying and thinking this thought.

When I teach this exercise in person, as the student is saying "the paper is blank", I interrupt them by saying things like "what am I going to eat later" or "I wonder what's on TV" or "I wonder if my friend will call". I say these comments just as they're starting to say the phrase "the paper is blank". They quickly realize how important it is to focus during this exercise.

I also teach that any object can work, such as a cup, as long as you adjust the sentence to "this cup is empty". For now, I want you to practice on the white blank paper while saying "the paper is blank". I will use this to add a special skill later in your training, and that and other future exercises will be difficult if you use a cup.

That said, using a cup and saying "the cup is empty" at other times will build strength. Later, I will teach you how to use the visual thought of the "blank white page" for strength like a force field. If you practice the exercise just as it is described, with no mental interference, I will be able to build on these teachings with future exercises like building blocks. If you modify it, the end result will not be as rewarding. You will not get the desired results to the degree that would otherwise be possible. Do not blame the chef if you don't follow the recipe he gives you!

Do this exercise three times a day or more for as long as you like. You can invoke this at any time, even while you are doing other activities, and especially when the paper is not physically in front of you. However, do it at least two times a day with a paper in front of you.

Other times, do this exercise only by visualizing it, as you would any other desired activity or job. Allow that to be the only exception for now, and use "the page is blank", visualizing the paper. You will find this to be a very liberating activity. In most cases, I have found rewards come quickly. No matter which exercise in this book you're doing, always do them every day.

Exercise 2: Open Window – Clear the Clouds

This is a 1-5-minute exercise you can/should do every morning and night. It will prepare you for future exercises, clear your mind, and bring attention to your inner self. It is the open window that begins your ability to communicate with yourself.

We will be using visualization, which is how you communicate with your intention. The purpose of intention is to communicate with your self. By putting your attention on this, your path becomes clear. The fog will slowly lift with continued exercise.

Not having clear intention creates fog. Just as thick fog is hard to see through, so it is with your ability or inability to hear your self and your correct intentions.

Be careful what you daydream about - you may receive it. Weigh it carefully to make sure it is what you want. Foresee its positive or negative consequences. If it is a true and positive need, then the following exercise will increase your ability to draw yourself to it. You must have a definite, practical plan of action to increase results. This shows your inner self that you are serious, and will encourage it to back you up.

Please take a moment to make a journal entry reflecting your thoughts so far. It will be interesting to you to reflect on them later when you have mastered this discipline.

Let's begin:

- Sit upright in a chair.

- Close your eyes.

- Visualize looking out of a large, open window at a blue sky on a warm summer day. (From this moment on, we will call any distractions "clouds".)

- The sky you are looking at is your clear, open mind. Do not resist the clouds. Allow them to pass. If you hold the clouds back, they will only pile up. If the clouds are too annoying, focus on your breath and imagine that your breath is the wind. Focus all of your mind's attention on every second of the slow breaths and physical movements of the body. Do not give any attention to the clouds. The clouds must move themselves with no help from you. Filling your mind completely gives the clouds no room to fit into or exist in your attention. This causes the clouds to move and leave your mind's vision.

- Fade from your breath back to your attention to the sky. If you give no attention to the clouds, they will float by.

Exploring Your Self

There is a part of everyone's self that is always watching and seeing the moment; that is, the moment things happen. It's almost as if it sees it happen before it happens. I have heard some martial artists describe seeing the path of a weapon and reacting seemingly before it actually happens. The person reacts through the self to in fact detect the path and allow the self to access the conscious, conditioned, trained response produced through repetitive training of his or her style.

The same is true of business training. Some businesspeople call this their immediate "gut sense". This course will train your conscious to react in a way that provides your self with choices regardless of the situation. In other words, you will no longer blindly react.

I have found that those who are in greater touch with the self through training use repetitive visualization to a reaction (or plan of action) to achieve a desired outcome in a physical or mental situation. Their execution is precise because their visualization was.

Some boxers use shadow boxing in their training, visualizing both an opponent's different attacks and their conscious, physical reactions. This tells the self what they want. There are others who merely visualize without physical movement and achieve results beyond belief.

As mentioned previously, in the days when people traveled by horse and carriage, they often put blinders on the horses. These were objects that were attached to a rope or leather harness to block the horses' view of their surroundings to prevent them from being startled and rearing up because of sudden movements on either side of them. The horses were allowed to see only the path in front of them. In life, many of us have been brought up with blinders on. Some say infants see and interpret more of the world around them than older children and adults do, but they lose that ability as they acclimate to society and its paradigms, until there's an illusion of walls that don't exist.

If our parents knew only one language and taught us only that language, naturally, we would have blinders on to all the other languages of the world. Our Inner Servant Self is like a horse with blinders on, capable of great strength, grace, and speed, but only able to see the road at its feet. We only see what we have been taught to see, and what the world expects us to see. (Our paradigm.)

You may be reading this book because you have gone through life feeling there is more without being able to see or feel it. A horse with blinders can still hear what's next to it, but can't see to react. I am glad you are hearing these words. Now let's work on removing those pesky blinders.

Goals:

- Write down a journal thought.

- To see one and maintain focus on all.

- To see all in one.

- To be in the moment as it unfolds.

Something to reflect on:

As we grow from infancy to adulthood, we tend to emulate our parents and other people in our sphere of influence. We adopt the accepted communication of the world around us - not just the spoken language, but our total surroundings. If we don't have a common perception of the parameters of the world around us, we can't communicate effectively with others. But, through training, we can see everything around us and all we're capable of doing physically and mentally. With a focused, open mind, small steps can unlock volumes.

Again, we are brought up to see only what we are able to see in the society we are accidentally born into, but our eyes are naturally meant to see more. The goal, therefore, is to open your eyes to see everything in your sight while focusing on an object or activity of interest. (That's what that blank paper exercise was about.)

Zone 1 – The Wall

Exercise 3 – Expanding Vision

This exercise will have three zones, and will be combined with exercises in later chapters. Practice it twice daily, while sitting down. This time can be set at your own liberty, based on your own progress. The purpose of this exercise is to maintain focus as a whole by focusing on the spot at the center of your vision.

- Sit in a chair about three feet away from the wall.

- Mark or find a spot on the wall in front of you.

- Without losing sight of that spot, look around it, expanding outward to the outermost parameters of your vision. At first, you may find your attention leaving the spot and drifting elsewhere. If so, reduce the size of the perimeter and keep your full attention on the center spot.

Journal thought: Write down your thoughts regarding your current training and the following thought: To look inward is to look outward. The world is a reflection of what we look for. Therefore, what we search for is already within us.

Zone 2 – Focus and Field

Exercise 4 – The TV and Everything Else

This exercise is to be done throughout the day, in your free moments. It is a mental exercise requiring ongoing practice. The goal is perpetual/unending growth, and the belief that you can always get better.

Throughout your day, while you're watching TV, and without looking away from the TV, also see and hear everything else around the room that is in your field of vision. At first, you may feel as though you are giving attention to one and then the other, back and forth, but with practice, you will see both. This will help make the self aware of your attention to all your surroundings, even if you're involved in another situation.

In martial arts, this is sometimes called "spatial awareness". When people are excited or scared, they tend to get tunnel vision, so they don't see or hear something coming at them from the sides or rear. If practiced enough, this will be like driving or riding a bike; you will do everything at once, unthinkingly. The TV exercise is just one way to practice it. You can concentrate on any object, anywhere, throughout the day. Focus on it while seeing and hearing everything around you. This exercise will help increase your reaction time to any situation.

Zone 1 is similar to Zone 2, but must be viewed and thought of differently as separate exercises to truly achieve the progress you want.

In your Goal Journal, write down and reflect upon the following thoughts:

To see what's really happening beyond the telegraphed movement, and to interpret upcoming events or danger, one must include all senses.

With a genuine need, unforeseeable events may make you aware of a pending event, allowing you to take appropriate action. This ability becomes stronger when we awaken ourselves from within.

Seeing what is really happening is simple to say but not easily done to the untrained. There are a few obstacles that are inherited in all of us to some degree.

Seeing everything in a conflict includes the ability to see what the other person is showing us and what he/she is not showing us. Humans have a tendency to fill in the blanks to define what they are not showing us, which is undoubtedly interpreted by one's personal experiences. That is, our personal blinders. Most of the time, we think faster than we interpret.

Wouldn't it be great to see what's really happening and react as though we were psychic? Read on . . .

Zone 3 - The Pebbles on the Table

Exercise 5 - Touch and Go

- Sit at a table.

- Place three objects in front of you at about an arm's length.

- Reach out and touch each one, looking at each as you do. Do this for the first three minutes. (Later, you may shorten this step to one minute.)

- Look at each object one at a time. Touch each of them, then look beyond them.

- Close your eyes and touch each of them.

- Open your eyes and alternate your action.

- Each week, add one more object. When your eyes are closed, visualize that picture in front of you.

Exercise 6 – The Forest

When done regularly, the following exercise is very rewarding and communicates to the self the need to observe. You will be surprised about what happens after a few weeks.

- The traditional exercise is to pick a young tree with leaves.

- Stand or sit in front of the tree and do the touch-and-go exercise. You will see that working with a living plant gives surprising results.

Bonus exercise

As you enter a room, close your eyes and count how many people you see. You may blink and look down so as not to draw attention.

NOTE:

These odd, simple exercises are part of a special recipe that I am using to create something very empowering and wondrous within you. At times, you may feel like Daniel in the movie *The Karate Kid*, painting a fence, taught to do it a certain way, but not understanding the connection. The point is to allow the teacher to work with you to achieve some fantastic results, using the teacher's talents to install new skills or awareness in a way that creates the least amount of resistance.

Throughout the centuries, our elders used stories to convey knowledge and stimulate thought. For these purposes, part two of this book contains a tale that illustrates the exercises and lessons you have learned so far, and more.

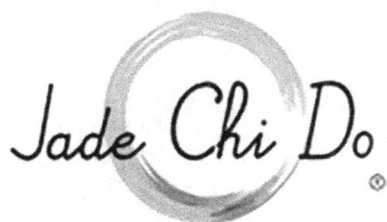

Jade Chi Do

PART II

Mastering the Warm Life Force for Life (and Love)

Jade Chi Do

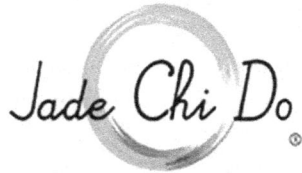

PART II - CHAPTER 1

The Adventure In Discovery Begins

There once was a young man named Abraxas who went through his life always feeling different. He knew he was a warrior because he had mastered many martial art styles. He also excelled in the sports of his day, the schools he attended, and even as a businessman. But even with all this success, and knowing what he had learned was good, he couldn't shake the feeling that there was more. There seemed to be something missing but he couldn't put his finger on exactly what it was.

Abraxas was walking down the street one day when he saw a shopkeeper putting a "help wanted" sign in his window. He needed work so he walked in to inquire about the job. The shop was full of statues, lanterns, vases, and a variety of odd objects, some old and some new. He thought, *This must be a buy, trade, or swap shop.* He walked to the back and found the shopkeeper, an old man with a thin, long beard like a wizard's, wearing a long blue coat with gold fringe tightly bound around its edges. He saw Abraxas approaching, and without looking up, said, "Did you come for the job, boy?"

Surprised, Abraxas answered yes.

"What's your name?"

"It is Abraxas. My friends call me Brax. What's yours?"

"You may call me Master Talon. When can you start, Brax?"

"What is required of me?"

"You must clean and dust the shop and every item in it each day, without missing a single one. You may start tomorrow, a half-hour after sunrise."

Brax agreed and left the shop thinking how great it was that he had a new job, but he was a little confused about why he had to be there so early.

The next day, he had to push himself to get out of bed. He liked working in the evening more. He had even scheduled his martial arts class in the evening. As he walked to the shop, he noticed a person walking out of it who seemed to vanish into thin air the moment he blinked.

He walked into the shop. As usual, Master Talon was waiting in the back room.

"Master Talon? I'm here!" he yelled.

Master Talon came out and handed him some rags. "Here you go, Brax. Remember, don't miss a spot."

As the weeks went by, Brax noticed that very few people bought, swapped, or traded. To entertain himself as he worked, he gave each piece in the shop a name. Each morning when he arrived at work, he noticed the pieces had been moved to different places. He also noticed that many martial art masters of great stature visited the shop every day. They would bring a piece in, go to the backyard with master Talon for some time, then come out and swap it with another piece in the shop. Brax thought maybe Master Talon was polishing the items.

This went on for some time. Finally, Brax had to ask, "Master Talon, what are these masters doing? Why are they swapping pieces?"

"Brax! You finally asked!" he replied with a chuckle. "I teach them."

"But they are all masters of different styles, and most hold the highest ranks. Why do they come to you?"

"Brax, do you recognize a warrior by sight alone?"

"No, Master Talon. It's a feeling I get. When I'm teaching martial arts, I sense those with greater capabilities in the class even before they become masters."

"Very good!" Master Talon said.

"It is like a glow without the light. I also feel those with even greater potential around me, but I see them surrounded by different kinds of light. Master Talon, will you teach me?"

"You have already started," said Master Talon. "But now is the time for you to formally accept this work. It will not be easy and it will require monotonous toil."

"I *am* ready!" Brax exclaimed. "I feel like I have waited for this for a long time without knowing I was."

"I know," said Master Talon. "Many pupils say to me it is a feeling that there is something more, and a feeling of waiting but not knowing what they are waiting for."

"That's it! Exactly what I have felt!" Brax said.

"You will start tomorrow. Now go home early, and when you come back tomorrow, bring me a dried ear of corn."

Brax opened his mouth to start asking the obvious question but the master held up his hand and said, "All will be revealed. The first thing you must learn is patience."

Brax smiled, said goodnight, and left.

As he was heading home, he thought this would be easy because he had mastered so many styles. He remembered all the great masters he had seen visiting Master Talon regularly and wondered why he hadn't figured out the master's role earlier.

The next day, Brax came into the shop early - an hour before daylight rather than only a half-hour - thinking he would catch the master sleeping. But as he walked in, Master Talon was waiting, sitting in a chair right in the middle of the shop, as if he knew Brax would be early.

"Brax, did you bring me the ear of corn with the dried kernels still on it?"

"Yes, Master Talon."

"Follow me."

They both walked into the rear courtyard. Master Talon took the corn from Brax.

"We will set it under this little roof."

There was a large stone with two boards rising from it. The boards had a seat around them and a roof on top.

"Before you start, Master Talon, I have no money to give you. How will I pay you?"

Master Talon answered, "For your first lesson, grab one kernel from the corn and give it to me. Your lesson shall be in this number, and this is your payment."

Brax was puzzled but did as he was told.

"Now sit down," Master Talon said. Brax did so.

"I need you to listen to me without thinking ahead of my speech. Even though many things will be similar to what you may think you know, don't let your cup be full."

"I won't, Master."

"Look at the sky. What do you see?"

"I see clouds being moved along by the wind."

"This week, look at the sky but see your mind's eye as the sky, your breath as the wind, and your concerned thoughts of today, yesterday, and tomorrow as the clouds. Now, what would happen, Brax, if all those passing clouds you see could not pass by?"

"They would be blocked and the sky would not be as peaceful to watch."

"Good," the master nodded. "The same happens if the clouds get backed up in the sky of your mind. Remember, the wind is what pushes the clouds past, and your breath is your wind, so focus on your breath with full attention and the clouds will pass. Then you will be in your sky of intention, with no distracting thoughts, seeing the moment as it unfolds. I eventually want you to do this morning and night, but for now, only do it at the beginning and end of class."

Brax sat next to the corn cob the master had set down. He closed his eyes to practice this new exercise, but his thoughts were wild in his mind. He quickly realized how much he would need to practice, for just when he thought he was not thinking, he found Master Talon's words repeating in his mind. After ten minutes passed, he went over to Master Talon.

"Master, I am finished, but this is hard. Do you have an exercise to help my progress?"

"Yes, and this is today's final lesson," said Master Talon. "To increase your progress, I want you to do this exercise just before you fully wake in the morning."

"Okay," Brax said eagerly. "Do you mean the time when I still feel like I'm asleep but I'm having my first thoughts of the day?"

"Exactly. Do the meditation exercise I taught you each morning for about ten minutes. When doing this, do not allow yourself to fall back asleep. This will strengthen your normal meditation with focus." Master Talon said this with a firm voice. Brax agreed and went home for the day.

Further into the moment

Journal Thoughts:

See what is there, not what you anticipate or assume.

See what is happening, not what you want to happen. (Not to be confused with visualization.)

Interpret not what is seen, but what is really happening.

Have clear intention of your needs.

Knock on the door of your inner self.

Your serving self awaits your clear communication and will listen.

The moment between sleep and wakefulness is a powerful space for communication. It is the best time to remember your dreams before they evaporate forever. This is the time when you can feed your intentions to your self. (This is a form of visualization. When you become aware of it, the meditative exercises written in this book will become gradually easier. Follow the exercises in order to achieve greater results. All results are cumulative!)

Brax woke up the next morning and practiced what master Talon taught him. As he walked to work, he noticed how beautiful the sunrise was. The golden sunlight splintering through the trees had a greater brilliance than he could ever remember seeing. The flowers seemed more colorful than ever too. It was as if he could see more clearly.

On these warm summer mornings, Brax walked by a small lake on his way to work. The cart path he walked along came within ten feet of the water's edge. On this particular morning, he noticed a young lady around his age standing by the water. She was casting a net into the water, attached to a rope she held. The rope went to the middle of the circular net, and as she pulled it in, the net would close.

He walked up to her and said, "Hello! My name is Brax. What's yours?"

"I am Lotus," she answered.

"What are you doing?"

"I am fishing for my father. He has gone to bring a vase to Master Talon."

"Your father must be a martial artist," Brax said.

"Yes, he is, but he is also a great businessman. He is the owner of The Cat's Claw Restaurant in the next town over."

"Why does your father have you fish here?" Brax asked.

"It's a special thing my father has me do for him. This lake has many fish along the shore. I cast this big net into the water and it sinks very slowly - so slow that the small fish don't move. The sides sink faster as the middle floats slightly. This makes a dome at the bottom that the fish get caught in without realizing they are captured. I then pull the rope slowly and it draws the sides in, capturing the fish. My father learned this from Master Talon. He told me this is one of the most precious lessons he ever received from him."

Brax decided to keep it to himself that Master Talon was his employer.

"That's very interesting. I'd like to stay and talk but I don't want to be late to work. I do hope to see you again, though," Brax said.

"I hope so!" Lotus said!"

As he walked away, he noticed the net she pulled in was full of fish and thought, "What lesson is this? How to *fish*?" He decided to ask Master Talon about it when he arrived at work.

As he got close to the shop, as usual, he saw a person leaving with a vase. This time he thought, "I know something about one of these masters that Master Talon instructs. That must be Lotus's father."

Brax walked faster so he could say hello, but he was too late. As Brax watched him walk away, he noticed something strange . . . the movement of his legs did not match the speed with which he was moving. He could not see his feet, for the grass was too high on the side of the path that led to the town. As Brax continued to study him, it seemed that his legs were walking at a slow pace, but his speed was much faster - about double what it should have been, like a fast jog or a slow running pace. This did not make sense to him. Naturally, he was full of questions for Master Talon.

As he entered, he saw Master Talon standing in the doorway at the back of the shop. They exchanged greetings and Brax got started with his work dusting and cleaning the shelf items. As the day went on, he couldn't wait for his lesson with Master Talon. He was trying to figure out how to ask him about Lotus and the net earlier that day. He had his ear of dried corn in an attached leather case he had sewn together to hold it securely on his belt. Some kernels were missing from the lessons Master Talon had already given him. He had found some lessons to be a little slow or simple, and he was worried he would use up all his corn kernels without being given the fishing net lesson Lotus told him Master Talon had given her father. Brax was very anxious but could not ask about it, as he was taught not to direct a lesson but to listen and act only upon what he was taught.

Finally, Master Talon called Brax to the back and asked him to bring some tea. When he brought it in, the master asked him to join him for a cup. Brax was excited because this was the first time Master Talon had invited him for afternoon tea. He thought, "Perhaps I can ask him about the net without losing a kernel. I'll casually bring it up."

He sat down across from Master Talon.

"The tea is good," Master Talon said. He then studied Brax for a few moments before saying, "I feel your attention has not been focused on your work as I have taught you. Is there something on your mind?"

So much for slipping his question casually into the conversation. Master Talon was one step ahead of him, as usual.

"Master Talon, may I ask you something? It's about something that happened to me on the way to work this morning."

Master Talon nodded.

"I met a girl halfway down the path. Her name was Lotus. She was fishing with a strange net. She said you gave her father a lesson about it."

"Ah, yes. The net. That is not only one lesson but many! It is also a philosophy, partially. Normally, I would have waited until you completed more lessons, and until I saw that they were taking effect within you from diligent practice. But since the seed of the net lesson was planted today, I will add it at the end of your normal lessons, with a warning - you will not benefit from it completely until you practice and begin to receive your current and past lessons. To skip even one lesson would increase the likelihood that you would lose out on the power of future lessons, and they will not give you all the results you desire."

Brax nodded in understanding. He wanted to get started right away but Master Talon said, "Now, I need you to go to the town and pick up a sack of grain. Master Blade, Lotus' father, is one of my pupils, and he's giving me this grain for his lessons."

"Where do I go?" Brax asked, disappointed.

"Go to the back door of The Cat's Claw restaurant and ask for him. Tell him I sent you so there would be no need for him to bring it."

"Okay. Do you want me to go now?" Brax asked.

"Yes. You'll need to be back before your lesson time. Now listen - this is important - you must carry this sack of grain with no cart. Put it on top of your back so there's one corner on each shoulder behind your neck. Keep your back straight. Do not hunch or bend forward. At the same time, walk a normal speed but put a very small spring upward in each of your steps. As you walk, count each step to fifty. When you reach the fiftieth step, put both legs together and jump up only one foot into the air. Do this for the entire walk. Look forward and see in front of you. At the same time, see around you. Also listen to all the sounds around you. Visualize that you are observing this all from just above yourself."

Brax then said, "Why see myself from above, Master Talon, may I ask?"

"You need to reach beyond yourself. I call it *seeing the sea around you*. It is a good time to do this because you will have a good anchor - the sack of heavy grain."

Brax was inching toward the door, anxious to be on his way.

"Oh, before you leave, Brax - could you get the vase on top of the high shelf outside?"

"Okay."

"One thing - you must keep both legs together and jump upward to grab it."

Brax nodded, confused, then went outside. He saw the vase and jumped up a few times but was about two feet short of reaching it. Frustrated, he went back into the shop and said, "Master Talon, can I get a ladder?"

"No, there's no time. You can get it for me later. You must leave so you will be back before dark."

"Okay, I will leave now," Brax said.

Brax was still confused but knew this lesson was related to the question he had asked. He had also done enough teaching to know that it was too early in his training for him to appreciate the lesson completely.

Brax arrived at the Cat's Claw restaurant, walked between two buildings along a very narrow, dead-end alley, found the back door and knocked. There was just enough room for the door to open. He moved to the side so the door wouldn't hit him, and so he could be seen by the person opening it. An elderly woman greeted him.

"May I help you, young man?"

"Hello. I'm here to pick up the large sack of grain. Master Talon sent me."

"Of course," the woman said.

"May I ask why the door opens outward in such a tight alley?"

"The door opens fully, as you see, and becomes a door for all," the old lady replied. "Master Blade uses this space for his meditation and privacy. He calls it his anchor space."

"I didn't mean to pry; I just was curious," Brax said.

She smiled and said, "Without questions, we would have no answers. Now wait here and I will get what you seek."

Brax thanked her, and as he looked into the restaurant, he caught a glimpse of Lotus. She turned to him the moment his eye and attention focused on her, then quickly walked over to him.

"Why are you here? I mean, it is nice to see you, but I am surprised!"

"Master Talon sent me to get a sack of grain from your father."

"Oh, I see. My father has always brought all the supplies to Master Talon. This is new."

As they were talking, the old lady returned with the sack of grain on a small, wheeled cart.

"Off to work, young Lotus,"she said.

"This is Tessa, my grandmother," Lotus said. "I must go."

"I hope we meet again," Brax said.

Over her shoulder while walking away, Lotus said, "May you have a safe trip back. Goodbye!"

Brax took the sack of grain off the cart and put it on his shoulders the way Master Talon had instructed him to, said goodbye to Lotus's grandmother, and went on his way. He counted his steps and put a small spring in each one. At fifty steps, he put his feet together and jumped up a foot, then did it again.

Then a new challenge arose. Brax thought, *How do I count while I listen to all of the nature around me and imagine myself watching me from above?* It sounded so easy until he had to count. Then he thought, *Hmm, I must apply the lessons I have learned.* He used the meditation technique Master Talon had taught him. As he was counting, after several jumps, he was able to do all he had been instructed to do.

Brax found counting to be his center; this enabled him to see all points around him. He looked in front of himself with his full vision, listened to nature's sounds, and imagined floating above himself and looking down. After a short time, he did not have to imagine anymore; everything happened at once. As soon as he noticed he was in this zone, his focus changed and he popped out of it. As thoughts came into his mind, he treated them as clouds and let them pass, and his counting was the wind, for now. As Brax walked along the path in a deep zone of this exercise, a sensation of peace stronger than he had ever felt flooded through him.

Suddenly, as if out of nowhere, a bandit jumped in front of him to attack him and take his grain. Without thinking, Brax jumped up and kicked him in the chest, as if he knew he was going to attack several moments before it happened. His kick was so precise, it knocked the wind out of the bandit and sent him sliding along the ground. He tried to get up but could only crawl. Surprised, he cried out, "Don't hurt me anymore! I'll leave! I'm sorry! I won't bother you again!"

Brax was surprised at the speed, precision, and unexpected nature of his reaction. He said, "Be gone! And think twice before you ever do something like this again!"

The bandit thanked him and crawled away on his hands and knees. Brax went on his way. He was so excited by what had happened, it took him a little while to resume his training. He thought of Lotus and hoped to see her again.

He started his training again and soon was at the entrance to Master Talon's shop. He went through the shop to the back and brought the sack of grain to Master Talon.

"Hello, Brax. I see you're right on time," Master Talon said. "Put the grain in the kitchen." Brax did so and returned to Master Talon.

"Is it time for my lesson, Master?"

Master Talon nodded yes. Brax handed him his ear of corn. He was going to tell him about the day's events and ask a few questions, but Master Talon had something else in mind. He took one kernel off the dried corn cob and handed it back to Brax.

"Now, go stand before the shelf, jump, and get that vase for me."

"I'm a little too short to reach it. I need a ladder. May I go get one?" Brax asked.

"No. Just do as I ask. Did you do the exercise I asked you to do on the way back from town?"

"Yes, Master Talon."

Stand in front of it and look at the object you wish to grab. See yourself grabbing it. Take two jumps - the first quick and short; and on the second jump, allow the release to send you where you wish to be."

Brax went outside and stood in front of the high shelf again. He put his feet together and jumped the way he was told to. This time, he surprised himself by jumping high enough to grab the vase! He felt as if he was floating for a second. He took the vase and landed on the ground, shocked at how easy it was compared to before. The jump felt more mental than physical, as if he had pushed his mind more than his body.

"How did I do that, Master Talon?"

"My dear Brax," Master Talon smiled. "Jumping while carrying the heavy sack of grain freed your body from the limits it had put on itself. Your mind too. Now, do you think you can grab the next highest vase?"

Brax then tried but couldn't, even though it was not much higher than the other one he had just grabbed.

"It's too high," Brax said.

Master Talon walked to where Brax was standing when he jumped.

"Watch me."

He jumped up and gracefully grabbed the vase.

Brax thought, *How can he jump higher than me, as old as he is?*

Master Talon said, "I will put it back." He then jumped and set it back gracefully. "I want you to do the same, now that you know an old man can do this."

Brax stood motionless for a moment, weighing the challenge.

"Do you not think you can?" Master Talon asked with a mischievous look.

"Okay, I'll do it," Brax said, feigning confidence. Inside, though, he felt doubt. But then he thought, *If Master Talon can do this, surely I can!* He jumped and grabbed the vase - not as gracefully, but he landed on the ground with it in his hand.

"Now, put it aside and come over here to meditate," said Master Talon, smiling.

Brax did so and sat down.

"Now that your lesson is done today, let's talk. How was your trip? Any obstacles?"

Brax hesitated to tell Master Talon about the bandit, fearing he would not send him next time. He did not want that to happen, mainly because he wanted to see Lotus again. In the end, though, he did decide to tell him since he brought it up. It didn't feel right to lie to him.

"Yes, there was a bandit, but I was deep in the exercise you told me to do so I reacted and deactivated him before I knew what I had done."

"Interesting," Master Talon said.

He was so wounded, he crawled away," Brax added.

"Your awareness and training is coming along well. Before I continue tonight's lesson, do you have any questions?"

"Yes," Brax said. "How is it I could jump so high?"

"Your body has natural limits and conditioned limits. Conditioned limits can be raised by training the body to go beyond them without letting it know. In many cases, this is the best way to train. It requires doing some exercises that seem to have nothing at all to do with the goal you seek. But a teacher uses this to build upon, and to get the trainee's attention out of the way to help them reach their goal. It is better to bypass your mind's resistance."

"Okay," Brax said, "Now I understand about the steps and the grain sack. Thank you. May I ask one more question?"

"Of course."

"I know now how I was able to jump and grab the first vase when I came back from town today. It was the lesson you had me practice while walking back. But how was I able to grab the second vase when I hadn't yet tried jumping that high?"

"Listen, Brax. This is very important. Remember when you watched me grab the higher vase?"

"Yes," said Brax.

"Remember this, because it will be part of your future lessons. Your mind either defines or fuels your perimeters or restrictions - the barriers or walls that you can or can't pass. Therefore, one can be set free from the wall by seeing another pass through its illusion of being there."

As Brax pondered this, Master Talon said, "Now to our meditation lesson. Close your eyes and tell me what you hear."

"I hear the birds," said Brax.

"Yes. What else do you hear?"

Brax was silent for a few moments when Master Talon asked, "What is hitting your body right now?"

"Oh, I didn't even hear it. It's the wind," Brax said.

"Now, while your eyes are closed, I want you to touch the tip of your nose on the right side with your right pointer finger while pointing to the sky with your other hand. Keep your arm close to your body. Do this now."

Brax did as he was instructed.

"Now, as you keep touching your finger on your nose in that position, open your eyes."

Brax opened his eyes.

"Do you see the tip of your finger?"

"No!" Brax replied, surprised.

"Now move your finger just a little closer to your nose."

Brax did and was surprised again. His fingertip appeared.

"I should see it just a bit out too?" he asked.

"Now put the finger back with both eyes open. You will see your finger."

"I do!" said Brax.

"Now take your finger away. Do you see your nose?"

"No," Brax answered.

"Your inner self - your mind - blocks this out so as not to distract you. Can you imagine staring at your nose all the time? We do but our self allows us to not see it, and to only see what is ahead of us so we won't be distracted. Now, close one eye and look at the other one and you will see the side of your nose."

"Wow! I never realized this," Brax said.

"Now, to tie today's lesson together – you did not hear the wind because it was not important, and your mind saw this because that was what you wanted. With your eyes and mind, your inner servant self blocks out anything that you deem unimportant, but also things that you were taught from birth do not fit into your surrounding world. Your paradigm. Our ability to communicate what we see, hear, feel, and smell in this spectrum - these are the common things around us. Our paradigm binds us. Now, this lesson will have two parts. If you work toward seeing things at their inception, you will be able to react to it in your conditioned way. This is imperative for success."

"Here's the second part of today's lesson. I know I'm giving you a lot to think about, but I feel you are ready for a jump, literally and figuratively."

Brax realized he was talking about the vase and laughed.

"As you get close to the inception, you will see that there are more things happening around you that you may not have seen or thought possible before. As long as you are anchored to your paradigm, you will be able to expand it and achieve great abilities in all aspects. Your training is going well."

Brax was a little confused, but he was able to see that his body as a whole – his eyes, sense of touch, and hearing filtered out a lot that he did not know. So, thinking out loud, he said, "This is why you include mind exercises with my physical ones - to achieve open awareness of more things around me in this world, and to learn about more that is available to me in this world, but that I do not yet see?"

"Yes, Brax, and how you see and interpret your present world equals our current paradigm only in part. Our training will expand the world around us and discover the fringe of the world in which we live. We will then reach beyond it to affect our world in a positive way. We will need to protect it soon. For now, when I say paradigm, I mean how you and most people see, communicate, and interpret the world around you."

"First, train to see the world around you in little steps. This will lead up to seeing it fully. Moving outward from this point will be very rewarding. Your ability will grow through these exercises I give you, and through the ones that will branch out from continuing this training by yourself later. But first, we must expand the smaller version of this whole world that you have. That part is what we make small by ourselves and other influences - a little paradigm, in a way. We will start there. These blinders must be lifted to reach the outer extremities of our world - to be able to reach beyond - and when anchored, we can pull from outer fringes of this world to affect our current world. That is, our current paradigm."

"I'm a little confused," Brax said. "Can you tell me more about our paradigm?"

"For now, our paradigm means how people and the whole world interact and communicate," Master Talon said. "How the world talks to you, and how you talk to it. How you hear and feel the wind. How you smell the roses. How it communicates its thorns to you. How you walk on the ground and feel the impact. How people talk to you, and all the ways you communicate back to them. Further, it is the board on which the game is played; our backdrop. Without this common variable, we as beings could not interact with this world, and we would all be lost to each other. A picture of our paradigm is that it's always moving forward, and always changing slightly, unnoticeably. We will be there to help it grow just like farmers who tend the fields. Does this answer your question, Brax?"

"Yes, in part," Brax replied. "So, I will understand more as I become more aware?"

"Yes. Understanding does not usually happen overnight; it happens by finding a good teacher, by training with sincerity, by persevering, and by embracing confusion as the doorway to knowledge. Abilities and enlightenment are the reward."

They exchanged a smile.

"It is getting late. You have had a full day today. Think about our talk on the way home. Your lesson is done."

"Okay, but what is my exercise to finish today?" Brax asked.

"What have you learned today, at least partially?"

"I have learned that my body can do more by doing an exercise that may seem unimportant. I have learned that exercises my body and mind can do that may or may not seem related can build cumulatively. At this time, I am the brick and the master teacher is the brick mason. It is not the wall but the structure it forms that makes it complete. Another thing I learned was being able to go past what I thought was my best. Seeing your example when you grabbed the vase taught me that my mind puts up many fake roadblocks that do not exist. So I see there are two ways to grow that equal one."

Well said!" Master Talon beamed. "You may go home. I will see you in the morning. Your exercise walking home will be to instruct yourself to listen, and to try to see and hear more detail. Find things you didn't notice before. But you must keep your eyes looking forward and use your full vision as best you can. Keep distracted thoughts to a minimum. Use lesson two – the meditation exercise called **Open Window**. On your walk back into work in the morning, review what you noticed the night before. Find something you did not notice."

Brax then went home and did as he was instructed.

The next morning, while walking back to work, he started to review what he may not have noticed on his walk home the night before. To his surprise, he did notice more things he had missed.

"Ah, I know why!" he thought. "I'm only seeing new things on the path because I'm walking in the opposite direction." As he continued on, he also noticed morning songbirds. As he neared the lake, he saw that Lotus was there fishing again.

"Hello, Lotus! What a nice surprise it is to see you again!"

"Thank you!" she replied.

"What brings you here so early? Is your father seeing Master Talon again?"

"No, I am here to catch fish for the restaurant."

"Don't you buy your fish at the market in town?"

"Yes, and that reminds me . . . I am in need of your help."

"My help? I'd be happy to help you, of course, but why do you choose me?" Brax asked.

"My father had to leave to take care of his sister. She's sick. She lives many days away. He said he may be gone for a few months. My uncle has taken over while he's gone. I was sitting on the roof - I go there to meditate sometimes - and I heard him in the alley behind the restaurant so I looked and saw him take money and sell weapons to some men who are well-known thieves in the area. I heard a little of what they were saying and it seemed they were planning something. I'm afraid no one will listen to me and I don't dare tell anyone at the restaurant in case they may be connected to my uncle and his crimes. I could be hurt or killed. So I thought of you. They don't know you so I thought maybe you could ask Master Talon if you could work there as a dishwasher. You could be my inside person and watch out for me until my father returns."

"I will ask Master Talon," Brax said.

Jade Chi Do

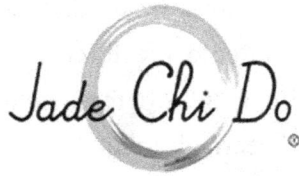

PART II - CHAPTER 2

The Difference

When he arrived at the shop the next morning, Brax asked, "Master Talon, may I take some time off to help Lotus? Her father is gone and she has some concerns about her uncle running the restaurant. She said something seems strange. She asked me to help her keep an eye on things."

"Is there a problem there?" asked Master Talon.

"I'm not sure, but I'll find out," Brax replied.

"Okay, you may," said Master Talon, "but keep me informed and stop in here just for your lesson days."

Brax was about to leave when Master Talon added, "Be careful of her uncle, Dakor. He teaches a very dark style that is based on cold life force."

Brax cringed. He understood what "dark style" meant but he was not familiar with the term "cold life force". Master Talon had never mentioned anything to him about it before. He assumed it meant "chi", a form of energy he had learned about from the other styles he had studied. So far, Master Talon had trained him to do ordinary exercises in a certain way, without telling or promising him any particular outcome; exercises that Master Talon promised would add up to something great, even without Brax knowing the outcome, or the theory behind the lessons. He wondered why he had never mentioned this to him before.

"Master Talon, what is cold life force?"

"Master Dakor, myself, and one other were students of a special teacher. To learn this style, we had to learn of this life force. It had two main sides - two opposites. Master Dakor decided to stay on the cold, dark side and practice its destructive effects. Still, we were like brothers; that is, until he killed our teacher and forever chose a path that lacks the light of life."

Brax had heard much about dark and light in his years of training, so he asked, "Master Talon, is this just good versus evil?"

"No, Brax, it's not that simple. Take the words good and evil out of it and all you're left with is a use of force that one connects and diverts within himself. One may use cold force to save a life. Is that not good?"

"Yes," said Brax.

"Brax, you must go one step further than that. It is not cold as in temperature. It is not like ice! The cold force is void of light because its core is void of love. Love at a deep level binds us all. This cold force is destructive to life, but warm life force is not. For example, a snake requires heat from other forces because mammals absorb and give out heat. Our cell energy of life is like light that radiates outward. We carry the lantern of light within us."

From his life experience, Brax figured he knew all about this life force, but Master Talon's words rang in his head, particularly his teaching to keep his mind like an empty cup and learn like a child without personal influence so he wouldn't miss the true lesson. So he asked, "Master Talon, what is *warm life force*? Is it just chi?"

"Brax, just is a big word. It's not just breaking bricks. This can be a cold force as well as a warm force. Let me ask you - what is your physical body made of?"

"Cells," answered Brax.

"What is the difference between a live cell and a dead cell?"

"Hmm . . . a form of electricity?" Brax asked.

"Would you say that without this, the cell has no life?" asked Master Talon.

"Yes."

"Would you say this is part of your life force of living?"

Brax answered yes again, then thought, *Wow! This is so much different than I thought it would be.*

"Brax, this life force is not here for you. It is here for you to use - like your breath uses oxygen. The blinders of our paradigm are like an eggshell. There are two basic ways to break it - from outside or from inside. Both achieve the result - a broken shell - but one way is destructive and the other is not. If it is broken from within, is there not something emerging that is much greater? So too is our warm lifeforce. We walk through life, and just as all our actions affect what we do and where we go, so our life force waits to be used further. There is a part of us that is mostly unused, like never taking a deep breath. You feel hints of it throughout your life, yet still it waits until one shows you it is possible; then your chains are released and you emerge from your shell. Master Dakor has chosen the use of the cold force, which is full of taking and very little giving, delivering disorder and destruction. Just remember, it has nothing to do with temperature."

"Thank you, Master Talon."

"Due to this recent event," Master Talon continued, "I am going to shift your lessons to a special training in the area of your awakening, and in directing this warm life force within you, to use in the world around you."

Brax was confused again but accepted it as the necessary passage to growth. He was eager to enter into a new phase of training.

"What is this next level called?" asked Brax.

"It is called **Jade Chi Do**. We have little time and much to cover. When would you like to begin?"

"With your approval, I will start tomorrow," Brax suggested. "Lotus said her uncle fired three of her father's workers at the Cat's Claw, and she wants me to start working there before he replaces them."

"Okay," said Master Talon. "I will meditate on your next lesson. We will start tomorrow morning before you go to work."

"Okay. Do you want me to do any of my duties for the shop before I go?"

"Not now. I'll see you in the morning. Goodnight."

Brax left the shop and went back to find Lotus to tell her the good news. When he arrived at the restaurant, many customers were dining. He found Lotus rushing back and forth between delivering food and washing dishes. She was visibly relieved when she saw him. She smiled and walked over excitedly.

"Can you start?" she asked.

"Yes, I can start tomorrow!"

"Great!" She smiled and gave him a quick hug. When they separated, he was captured by her eyes for a moment. Lotus was too busy to notice his smitten expression.

"As you know," she said, "most days, we're only open for lunch and dinner, so we start at eleven a.m. and go home at seven-thirty; sometimes later."

"Got it," Brax replied.

"My uncle isn't here right now. I'm so glad you're able to work here. You can fill in for one of the workers he fired."

"Why did he do that? asked Brax.

"I have no idea. It doesn't make any sense. They have been loyal employees for my father for a long time."

Lotus was called by a customer and excused herself. Brax sat and waited for the restaurant to close, then walked her home. The full moon along the path illuminated everything with an ethereal silver light.

"Lotus, may I ask, why is your uncle so odd?"

"My uncle has always been a little mad that my grandparents gave the restaurant to my father."

"Why?"

"He was adopted, so he may feel that's the reason they didn't give it to him. My grandparents said it was for other reasons, but never told me what they were."

They stopped to rest at the small pond where they first met. The water reflected the moon, flickering like a thousand tiny candles. Lotus walked to the edge and looked into the still water.

"It's like a mirror with a silver frame!" she said excitedly.

Brax looked at her reflection and was again taken aback by her beauty. The moonlight was doing its eternal magic, illuminating Brax's heart with its warm light even more brightly than the pond.

"Can I show you something my father showed me?" Lotus asked.

"Sure!"

"When the moon is full and the water is calm like this, he would tell me to find two flat stones the size of my palm."

Brax stood staring at her, waiting for her to continue the story.

"Well, go ahead, silly!" she said playfully.

"Oh, sorry!" Brax replied. He immediately began searching, found two perfect stones, and returned to Lotus. She asked him for one of them.

"Now, let's both stand thirty feet apart on the shoreline. Our goal is to skip the rocks along the top of the water, aiming for the middle of the pond, and we must throw our rocks at exactly the same time."

Brax agreed but was perplexed, wondering what the purpose was. He walked away along the side of the pond until he was thirty feet away from Lotus.

"Okay, I'm ready," Brax said.

"On the count of three!" Lotus said. "One . . . two . . . three!"

They both threw their stones and watched them skip along the water toward the center of the pond. The stones got closer and closer to each other before they finally stopped and sunk into the water. The ripples from each skip of the stones rippled outward across the pond in every direction.

"That was nice," Brax said, still confused about her reason for this game.

Lotus said, "Wait just a moment. Keep watching."

They watched the ripples, and as they touched each other and rippled back again, an amazing thing happened. All the ripples joined and multiplied until they illuminated the entire pond with sparkling, silver and gold light that was so brilliant, it reflected upward onto the trees surrounding the pond.

"Amazing!" Brax exclaimed. "I've never seen anything like it!"

"My father told me our thoughts and actions create reflections and ripple outward in the same way," Lotus added.

"Your father is very wise," Brax said. "Thank you for sharing this with me."

He felt there was an even deeper lesson to be learned from this, and knew that when he was ready, he would see it.

Jade Chi Do

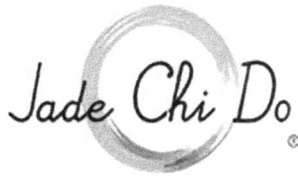

PART II - CHAPTER 3

Special Awareness: The Art of Invisibility

Before Brax went to his temporary job at the Cat's Claw restaurant, he headed to the shop for his morning training, as Master Talon had instructed him to do. As he walked along the path to Master Talon's shop that summer morning under a calm, blue sky, he passed a majestic maple tree on his left, not far from the shop. His thoughts were on his work and all the ways he might help Lotus at the Cat's Claw.

As he walked by the tree, he heard a voice say, "Good morning, Brax!"

He stopped, thinking it was Master Talon. A chill came over him because he sounded so close. He slowly turned to look behind him and saw Master Talon sitting in a chair by the tree in plain view. Brax was confused because he remembered looking at the tree as he approached and passed it.

"Good morning," Brax replied. "How is it that I did not see you as I approached? How long were you there?"

"I have been sitting here meditating for the last two hours or so."

"Master Talon, I was looking right at the tree as I approached it. How is it that I did not see you?"

"Brax, today's lesson is best taught here." Master Talon stood up slowly and added, "Sit in this chair." Brax did so.

"What do you see?"

"I see the path I just walked," Brax answered.

"May I ask what you were thinking when you were walking toward the tree?"

"Many things. My mind was full of concerns about the situation with work and Lotus." "Did these thoughts solve anything?"

"No," admitted Brax.

"And you did not see me, right?"

"Right."

"Brax, if I live in the past, I may trip in the present. What then happens to the future?"

Brax thought for a moment and said, "I see. My future may not have the outcome I desire."

"Yes, but let's tie this into your lesson today," said Master Talon. "When someone is distracted with thoughts, they cannot see all that is around them. Crowded thoughts make it difficult or impossible to solve a problem. In most cases, they are distractions from achieving one's objectives. It is more than just being present in the moment, it is being present in the moment *and* aware of one's objectives and purpose."

"Okay, so don't think of anything, right?" Brax asked.

"Brax, you are thinking, but in this case, your thinking is observing without placing conscious thought to it, so this is the exercise I want to teach you. As you sit in the chair, tell me what you see."

Brax sat down.

"What is next to the big rock on the other side of the road?" asked Master Talon.

"Wow," said Brax, "I don't know. Is it another chair? I can't believe I didn't see that! Wait a minute . . . I know why I didn't see it when I was walking to the shop - because it's behind the rock, but looking back from where you were sitting, I can see it. I still have no idea why I didn't see it until you brought it to my attention, though."

"Ah, so the key is bringing it to your attention!" exclaimed Master Talon. "Sometimes, when we're focused on something inward - that is, within ourselves - or outward, like a person or object, we lose really being there, or what is really happening. Even when we read or listen, we may do the same. In a way, we are often unconsciously or consciously so focused on what we want to see, we do not see what is really there, with any of our senses. This also happens when we are distracted and unfocused; our self fills in the blanks of what we expect to see."

"I am projecting what I expect to see?" asked Brax.

"Yes. You also project to others your attention on them. In most cases, if another feels this, it doesn't matter. When you are teaching, learning, or connecting, it is healing and gives warm force. But projecting one's attention negatively can be harmful.

You may see now the need to be aware that this action is important in business, combat, or in your case, with your task of helping Lotus. For this reason, I must teach you in a special way. Most of your training so far has been with exercises to build up to something without allowing you to know the outcome so that your blinders do not impair your learning and you can gain access to the true abilities of the exercise. In this new training, I will go into the details a little more deeply because you may have some unique challenges coming up as a result of helping Lotus. Many successful people in all avenues of life, including business, acquire these skills to develop a strong focus, as well as an awareness of those who may not be acting in their interest. Master Dakor has refined this sense and is very aware. This heightened sensitivity is very strong in people with a powerful ability to focus. I know you don't want to let Lotus's uncle know you're there to help her, so to avoid creating suspicion and making her uncle aware of your true purpose, you must see yourself as an actual hired worker. You will be close to her uncle, and there may be times when you will be watching and observing his activities. To prevent being discovered or even noticed, we will now work on learning and becoming sensitive to this warm force. Are you ready?"

"Yes, Master Talon."

"Good. Here is the start of your lesson. Have you ever looked at someone who was unaware of you, then they turned and looked right back at you, as if they felt you watching them?

"Yes."

"They may not have known why, but they felt the projection of your focus on them. The reverse is also possible. To control your projection on another, one must watch and actually not be focused on the active thought of what they are watching. This may sound strange, but this is done by allowing your conscious mind to be occupied with seeing all around the object itself, as if you're looking out a window and just observing everything but nothing in particular. You must not think of the person you're watching. Also, you cannot think of the reason why you're doing that job when you're near Master Dakor. He will feel it. Brax, what has made you great at your styles and other endeavors may work against you when you help Lotus."

"Okay, but how do I train to not be felt by such a strong master as Dakor?" asked Brax nervously. "If I understand what you're saying, I must look at all that is around me yet recognize it and not apply thought to it?"

"Yes. You must know your objective internally. You must have a deeper focus other than on the person. Let's continue; there's not much time. Your exercise today is called **Blue Sky.** Stay there where I was sitting and look straight in front of you at that other chair you were just talking about, the one in front of the large stone across the path. As we continue, we will call that a *spot*. This way, you can practice anytime using any spot, like a cup or any other object, in the center of your vision."

Brax focused on the other chair as Master Talon continued.

"Look at it. Take a deep, full, silent breath through your nose; not too much chest movement. Expand your stomach outward when you inhale. Hold it for three seconds. At the peak of the full breath, exhale slowly with your mouth for about five seconds, pulling your stomach in. Now completely exhale and count to three before you repeat the exercise and inhale again. Do this twice, at least. Next, as you exhale, focus on the spot - in this case, the chair. As you do this, do not think of the chair; just see the chair. Next, expand to see your whole peripheral vision while continually seeing the spot in the center of your vision."

Brax kept practicing this. At first, he found that looking to the sides pulled him away from the center of the spot - the chair.

"I lose the center," he said.

"You lose the center because you are using your conscious mind to see it. Let your inner self know your goal and trust that it is watching."

"I will try that," said Brax. After a few moments, he exclaimed, "Wow, I see what you have described."

132

Just then, it started to rain rather heavily.

"Brax, continue this exercise and see the raindrops as they fall," said Master Talon.

Brax did so. All of a sudden, he shouted, "What?" then said, "Wow! This is amazing! Everything went into slow motion. I could see the drops as each one landed. It didn't last long, though. As soon as I noticed it, it stopped."

"Your conscious mind noticing is what interrupted you and took you out of the exercise. Normally, it takes much longer to attain this, but I am focusing my teaching upon you. I know you're ready. When you practice, you will find that you're able to see the chair and observe your surroundings even when walking or doing a task. By doing this, you'll be able to safely observe Master Dakor. You may need to divert your attention at first when you're in conversation with him or he may feel your intent. To avoid this, you must see a picture of something else in your mind, such as Lotus or some inanimate object. Until you improve, this will divert your true objective as you speak to or look at him."

Master Talon continued, "Another powerful technique is to see yourself looking back in the mirror with no thought. I was supposed to teach you all of this much later in your training, but again, due to the circumstances you will be faced with, we must accelerate your training. I know I have talked much more than I usually do with you. Do you have any questions?"

"Master Talon, my main worry is . . . will I be prepared?"

"Your choice and confidence with your training will be the seed that will enable you to succeed. We will continue your training of the warm life force. This will be imperative for you when you're near Master Dakor. All teachers have the ability to project their teachings to accelerate special students. That is my intention. Ask your inner self to do the work, not your conscious mind. When you're focused or thinking deeply with the conscious mind, you may not succeed. The objective must become a task of your inner self, not your conscious mind, to be strong enough within to succeed. In this case, I am sure you will be observing Master Dakor, so you will have to shift from *thinking what you want* to *seeing what you want*. You must keep your conscious mind in the act of observing - again, like looking through a window. The window becomes your conscious mind, and your inner self is the part that becomes the one looking out."

"Master Talon, you've given me much to figure out. To get this straight, as I sit in the chair now, I start the exercise by breathing the way you instructed. I begin to look at the chair across the path in front of the stone. Then, without thinking, I see all around it using my full vision. At the same time, I continue to look at the chair, understanding that even though I am looking at it, I give no conscious thought or attention to the chair. I just observe without defining or acknowledging it."

"That's right. This is a special exercise in communicating with your inner self, leaving your conscious mind without attention yet still reacting to your surroundings, meaning you could still move or react to a challenge should it happen."

"Why is this important?" Brax asked.

Our conscious mind is our broadcasting station and can be felt. Have you ever looked at someone and they turned back like they felt you looking? Or, you were standing and turned because you felt someone looking at you?"

"Yes, now that you mention it, that has happened to me many times, but I always just dismissed it. Is that what this exercise is about?"

"Yes, in part. It is a little more complicated than that, but you will grasp more in time. Do this exercise as much as you can to get a habit in place. This step is important because it opens an important communication within yourself. This will help accelerate your next lesson. It will activate awareness of energy from inside and outside yourself; energy that you may direct."

Brax said okay but was a little nervous because of this very intense and mysterious lesson. The concern for his safety he could hear in Master Talon's voice also put his nerves on edge.

"Master Talon, you mentioned a mirror. Were you in a mirror?"

"The mirror, yes. I am glad you asked. If I chose to be able to observe you and not to be noticed, there are certain things I would need to apply. I would apply no thought to that which I'm watching. I would wait for the time when the subject is in action and concerned with their activities. I would move with full attention, sending no thought. I would see myself looking at myself as if I'm in a mirror, in full detail; a full mirror image. At the same time, I would walk or observe my conscious mind making a loop. This mirror exercise

135

creates great stealth, which you will need, Brax. This last mirror exercise is something that, with practice, you can work up to. In reality, the more you practice, the faster it will evolve. Today's training will help you. The more you train, the greater your ability will become to work with that part of you that is able to help you. The future training exercises will come easier as well."

"Thank you, Master Talon," Brax said, feeling more relieved. "I will practice and meditate upon today's lesson."

"Good," Master Talon said. "To accelerate your training, today I want you to pay attention to things and spots around you. Give a few seconds to things that you normally wouldn't. This will help you with your presence in the present."

Brax trained for a little while longer, then went to the restaurant. When he arrived, he saw Lotus in the front, clearing dishes from some tables. She greeted him and said, "My uncle will be coming later today. Please keep your eyes open. I'm not sure who he's going to hire. I did tell him that I had hired you because I needed somebody right away. He seemed disappointed but said he wanted to meet you to approve your working here."

"Where do you wish me to start?" asked Brax.

"We need to sweep up the dining area. It has become dusty and dirty since the other workers were fired. I had no idea how much they did until they weren't here anymore. Please go and sweep the dining room, then do the dishes, then bring out the rubbish, then go refill the grain bins. My uncle will want to meet you late in the day."

"Okay," Brax said, a little concerned about meeting him. As he went to get the broom, he reflected on Master Talon's training earlier that day. If he was going to meet Master Dakor soon, he would need to start training right away and practicing the new skill Master Talon tried to teach him. It made him feel better to know that he had most of the day to practice. He was amazed at how quickly Master Talon was able to instill his training in him, and he looked forward to the next lesson.

As he started sweeping, he practiced the Blue Sky exercise, focusing on its main point of expanding around whatever "spot" he had chosen. As he swept, the spot he chose was the point where the broom met the floor. He also observed all around himself. He found that no matter what his task was, he could do this exercise by choosing a new spot.

As Lotus walked into the dining room, Brax noticed that he saw her walking in while he was practicing the exercise. It was amazing how he saw and felt her moving toward him.

He wondered why he had never felt like this before. He recalled the incident with the bandit on the road. If he had known this technique then, he wouldn't have even needed to kick him because he would have felt him approaching earlier. He did not fully understand this new teaching, but he knew that Master Talon's exercises always held more meaning than they appeared to on the surface, and that they always built into something even greater. He was happy he could feel results, which increased his confidence. He knew this was a very important seed that was going to help him succeed. As he worked and practiced through the day, he felt better about the upcoming meeting with Master Dakor.

Jade Chi Do

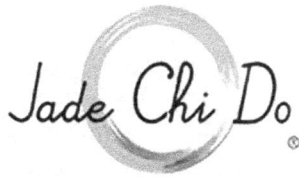

PART II - CHAPTER 4

The Emerald

As Brax was washing the last few dishes, almost through with his day's work, a cold chill shot up his spine. Then a voice sounded out, very close behind him.

"So you're Brax."

Without turning around, Brax answered yes. He raised his head slowly and took a special breath the way he was taught. He then reflected upon himself like a mirror and thought, "I am a dishwasher. I am looking at myself and seeing nothing but this." He then turned, and as he looked into Master Dakor's eyes, he felt as if he was pushed by just his presence. He also felt a kind of pressure emanating from his eyes.

"Hello, sir. Nice to meet you."

"So, you're the new person Lotus has hired?"

"Yes, sir. I was dining here and noticed how busy she was. I asked if she was short on help. It was very crowded that day."

Master Dakor looked at him for quite some time. Brax felt him waiting to feel more from him. He remembered Master Talon's teaching and concentrated even harder on looking at himself as if he were a mirror, looking right back at himself. It felt like a shield. No longer did he feel the pressure from Master Dakor. Then Brax said, "I must get back to my dishes, sir."

"I will be introducing you to the new employees tomorrow. Be sure to fill the grain bins before you leave today. We will talk more soon."

Master Dakor walked away. As Brax started washing the dishes again, he was amazed that the mirror lesson worked so strongly, and came out of him from a place of no thought, naturally, even instinctively. It was as if a part of him was defending itself.

Later in the day, Lotus walked over while Brax was filling the grain bin and said, "I overheard my uncle arranging a meeting with the same person I saw him with when I told you about the trouble that was happening. They will be meeting soon in the alley, right by our back entrance. I need you to listen from the roof. Can you do that?"

"Okay," said Brax. "How do I get up to the roof?"

"The fastest way is to go up near the back entrance in the alley because it's so narrow, you can touch both sides and walk yourself up, or there's a ladder on the other side of the restaurant you can use."

Brax chose the ladder because it was more concealed. When he was on the roof, he walked over by the rear entrance, then sat down and meditated as he waited for Master Dakor to show up for his meeting. As he sat there, he thought about how fortunate he was to have received this valuable training from Master Talon. If he hadn't, he would have been defenseless against Master Dakor's dark powers.

It was starting to get dark. Brax noticed lantern light coming from the alleyway below. He heard the kitchen door open and slam, then an unfamiliar voice said, "Did you get everything in place? Are you ready?"

He heard Master Dakor reply, "Not yet. A few obstacles just came up, but I intend to work on them in the next few days. I only have two of my people to use because my niece hired a new employee. I should be able to do what we planned, though. Are you ready?"

The other voice answered, "Yes. I'm at the cabin just inside the tree line outside this village, on the east path going out of town. I'll be waiting there. Are you sure you will be able to find out where the emerald is?"

"Yes, I am," Master Dakor replied.

When they left, Brax went back down the ladder. He found Lotus standing on the ground when he climbed down. She reached for his hand and he took it, not because he needed help, but because he wanted to feel her hand in his. She was well-named - her skin was as smooth as lotus petals. After being on the cold roof so long, the warmth of her touch was welcome too. He held her hand a little longer than he needed to, then let go, not wanting to be too forward. She smiled shyly, then asked him what he had heard her uncle say. Brax answered, "I'll walk you home. We can speak when we get further away from here."

They walked down the same path they used the previous evening. When they were near the south path, a good distance away from the Cat's Claw restaurant, he told her everything he had overheard, then asked, "What is this emerald he was talking about?"

"I don't know," Lotus replied. "It's so strange. Other than my uncle, the only person who might have known was my grandfather, but he has passed away. We can ask my grandmother, though. Hopefully she'll know."

"Okay. Can we do that tomorrow?"

"Yes, but it sounds like you're going to have a big day meeting the new people my uncle has hired. I haven't met them yet either."

As they continued along the path, he said, "I wanted to say thank you for skipping the stones on the pond with me yesterday, and for the story you told me about it. It was incredible to see the moonlight."

What Brax was really thinking was how incredible it was to see her beautiful face illuminated by the moonlight as she looked at the water, and how her hair and skin shone as magically as the pond had. He couldn't bring himself to say it, but his smitten expression told her everything he couldn't. The heart has its own way of speaking, and needs no words. She smiled, looked into his eyes, and said, "Thank you. It was very nice to be able to share that with you as well."

142

They continued walking quietly for a moment when she said, "I'm sorry I brought you into this task with the restaurant."

"Don't worry about it," Brax answered. "There's definitely something going on, and it sounds like even you are surprised about it, so we have a little mystery to unravel. I look forward to looking into that tomorrow."

When they arrived at Lotus's house, he told her he would be there in the morning. They said goodnight and he went on his way, full of questions about Master Dakor that he wished he could ask Master Talon, especially the strength of his presence that tried to overtake him when he stood in front of him. He couldn't wait for his next training session.

The next morning, Brax was walking down the path leading to Master Talon's shop.

He practiced the exercise, focusing on a spot as he was walking while paying attention to his peripheral vision, noticing things around him that he normally wouldn't see, from large objects all the way down to a bush or flower.

As he approached the same tree, he did not see his teacher or the chair, but when he was about ten paces before the tree, it was as if they suddenly appeared in the same place.

"Very good," said Master Talon.

"I'm surprised I didn't see you sooner, but I'm happy that I saw you before I actually walked by the tree," said Brax.

"Your practice is serving you well," said Master Talon.

"Thank you. You told me to keep you updated. I'm just a little worried. I do have a question about an emerald he appears to be looking for."

Master Talon considered this for a moment, then said, "I don't know about any emerald other than the Crown Prince Emerald. It is rumored that he had to give it to a trusted warrior for safekeeping because of enemies within his own ranks. It is very large and of great value. I can see why Master Dakor would want it. It will enable him to impose his cold force on many people. It is inevitable that you will be in direct conflict with him."

"This force I felt from him - what is it? And what must I do to defend myself?"

asked Brax.

"What you felt from him was the use of his force from his whole self. Many people have felt this. Have you ever been in a conversation with someone, and though they weren't angry or touching you in any way, you started to get a threatened feeling from them, as if they were pushing you?

"Yes."

"Since neither of us know when this conflict will occur, you must learn fast. I will tell you what you need to know about cold force. Please have a seat."

They both sat on the grass and Master Talon began. "Some feel very intimidated by people like that, but for those who master this powerful tool, the choice simply becomes which use of force they will use. Cold force can make a person cave in, attacking his inner confidence. It uses, feeds on, and is influenced by the use of power over those of low confidence who live in uncertainty. Master Dakor feeds on the intimidation and fear his energy causes in others. All beings that use cold force do. The truth you need to know is that they cannot take or control your power, though they would like you to believe they can, because that gives them the ability to feed upon your fear and intimidate you. Someone trained in the cold force can be very manipulative, playing on fears and its energies within others."

Brax listened carefully, knowing this information could save his life. Master Talon continued, "Again, neither cold force nor warm force are inherently evil or good. They are like a frequency of choice that can be creative or destructive. In many big, condensed cities, cold force is normal; a subconscious, defensive reaction. Some people are quick to explode in anger and tell you off. This emits a strong cold force energy, frequency, or vibration to mask themselves from those who feed on fear. They use the cold force to hide their insecurities. In short, those who use the cold force seek confidence outside of themselves by feeding off outside events that generate fear. The warm force seeks and emulates confidence from within, moving outward like sunlight sending shafts of light into darkness. Feeding this warm force is love, continuity, and overall harmony. The cold force is neither good nor evil. When one masters both, for example, he could use the cold force to save a life. Again, neither are based on good or evil, but the cold force is destructive by nature. This by itself does not help those around you. There are some, like Master Dakor, who have mastered a lot of the warm force and choose to direct it to the cold force, feeding on this to control others."

Master Talon paused, allowing Brax to absorb all this new information.

"I have spoken much about this now, Brax. I don't want to overcomplicate it, or make you have pre-judgments based upon what you've learned from prior activities. As you know, it is easier for someone to learn something wondrous if their self is not in the way. But in this case, because of your coming challenge, as I said, I must speed up your training. I as a teacher have the ability to help you in this acceleration."

"How may I be more aware of this - to be able to utilize this force?" asked Brax.

"This brings us to our next training," Master Talon replied. "The first thing to do is feel this warm force, which has always been hidden just under your senses.

Jade Chi Do

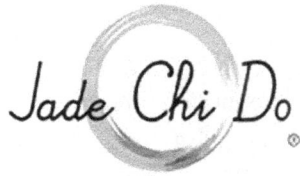

PART II - CHAPTER 5

Awakening

As Master Talon walked alongside Brax, they came to a field across from the pond. A tall birch tree stood in the middle of the field.

"Stop," Master Talon said. "We will do our lesson here."

They both walked into the field and Master Talon directed Brax to look at the maple tree.

"What do you see in front of you, Brax?"

"I see a tree in the middle of a field with no other trees around it."

"What else do you see?"

"I see that it's straight, its roots are in the ground, and its leaves reach up to the sky."

"Good," Master Talon replied. "If a tree grows in the middle of the forest and the rest of the forest is cut down, the tree is likely to fall when high winds come. It is better for the tree to be at the edge of the forest and experience some wind as it grows so its roots will grow deep and strong. Knowing this, what more can you tell me about this tree, being in the middle of this field?"

"By looking at this massive tree, I can see that it is well-rounded, tall, and straight. It must be deeply rooted because it has faced many storms over the years."

"Yes, Brax. Our lives are no different, so our choice *must* be to embrace adversity and never give up. The cold force would only look at the storms of life as a challenge to their power, a means of controlling them, not an instrument of development and growth. Do you understand?"

"Yes, Master Talon."

"Good. Your lesson starts now. As you observed, the tree is always reaching and aligning with gravity, and so too are we in this exercise. It is called **Heaven and Earth.** Just as the tree reaches to the heavens, it also roots deep within the earth. As you know, the leaves soak up the sun's energy. What else do we have in common with the tree?"

"The tree is made up of live cells, as we are. As you taught me, we are also connected by a unit of energy, like electricity - our life force. There can be no denying this."

"Yes, Brax," said Master Talon. "It is time to awaken that which has always awaited discovery within you. As you know, it gives everyone many hints over the course of a lifetime. Come. I want to show you something."

Master Talon started walking toward the tree. Brax followed. When they arrived, Master Talon said, "Stand facing the tree, about ten paces away from it, with your feet shoulder-width apart, arms down on your side."

Brax did so.

"Now look at the tree and imagine you are its reflection, as in a mirror. Allow that to be the only thing that occupies your conscious mind. Some refer to this part of the mind as the part that is thinking out loud or thinking to oneself. Today, I will teach you only one part of the six parts of this exercise. The first part of Heaven and Earth is something we call rooting. Inhale through your nose, filling your belly."

Brax again did as he was instructed.

"Good. Now lift your arms and hands like wings, no higher than midway, while bending your knees and sinking toward the ground, as you are inhaling. Next, start to stand up, unbending your knees while exhaling slowly through your mouth. At the same time, lower your arms until your palms are close to your sides. Do this slowly and work toward a non-breakage of movement, smooth and unending. I placed you in front of the tree to accelerate your training. Next, add visualization, connect your breath to your palms and your feet. When you breathe in, connect and visualize inhaling and exhaling from your feet and palms. Imagine you're still the mirror of the tree, engaging the warm life force that connects all."

As Brax did this, he said, "I feel a kind of pressure in my palms when I lower my arms, flowing through my legs to my feet. It's a little like the pressure I felt from Master Dakor. But this is a flowing feeling. The feeling I got from Master Dakor was a non-flowing feeling."

"That is very good, Brax. You must practice this as much as you can. To direct the warm life force, one must first root and connect. This will unlock the paradigm most are living under and the blinders it puts on them. This life force will also take on a real feeling, allowing you to actually feel it, just like you would feel any physical object. As it becomes tangible, you will be able to use and direct it. And because it was always there, it will manifest itself more and more. Again, this is just part of your lesson, but we must go further into something else because you're going to be meeting Master Dakor today.

"I am a little concerned about meeting him and his new hires. I have a strange feeling of dread," said Brax.

"Brax, you must embrace this situation. Imagine you are fishing with a weighted net.

You have cast the net just by working at the restaurant; now you must blend in. As the net falls, you cannot let on what your intentions are. The only way to handle Master Dakor is to embrace what I have been teaching you. That is how you will discover what they are planning."

Brax thanked Master Talon, practiced a little more, then left for the restaurant to work.

As Brax walked down the path, he noticed a man walking in front of him. Brax was walking a little faster so he caught up to him. As he was starting to pass the man, he said hello, then noticed something. He was the bandit who tried to rob him before. The bandit recognized Brax too. He quickly and nervously said hello in return.

"What brings you this way?" Brax asked.

"Since my encounter with you, I have not done that again and have been looking for regular work."

"What is your name?"

"I am Subdo. I'm going to work at the Cat's Claw restaurant. Master Dakor has hired me."

Brax felt a little angry but concealed it, remembering Master Talon's teaching that he is only to cast the net, not disturb the fish.

"I am working there also," said Brax.

As Brax looked into Subdo's eyes, he felt his force showing as it pushed upon him. Subdo became very intimidated and started looking down to hide his fear. Brax was amazed that he was sensitive to this but knew this ability must have come from his training.

As they neared the Cat's Claw restaurant, Brax saw Lotus at the front entrance and walked in that way so he could greet her. Subdo walked to the back-alley entrance where Master Dakor said he would meet him. Brax walked over to Lotus.

"Good morning, Brax!"

"Good morning! Did you talk to your grandmother?"

"No, I was waiting for you. Let's go ask her now. Master Dakor will be here in about thirty minutes."

Her grandmother was cleaning a table in the corner as they approached her.

"Grandma Tessa, I must ask you a question. Do you know what the emerald is? I heard my father mention it." She didn't mention her uncle because she didn't want to upset her, or tip off Master Dakor if he came back earlier than expected and overheard them talking. Her grandmother quickly sat down at the table she had been cleaning. She looked at Lotus and Brax and said, "Sit."

They looked at each other, a little surprised by her abruptness, then sat down.

"I am surprised you overheard him talking about this," she whispered. "Nonetheless, he was given a great task to watch over this emerald. It is the Crown Prince Emerald, one of the biggest in the world. Before the crown prince died in battle, he gave this to your father, the soldier he trusted most, because he feared it would fall into the wrong hands. It's immense value can give too much power to the wrong person. It is in a special spot known only to him. However, it seems rumors have gotten out."

"We won't say anything," Lotus said.

Lotus was shocked to learn that her father was the trusted warrior of the late crown prince. Customers were starting to come in so Lotus said, "I must go wait on them. Thank you, Grandma." Her grandmother returned to her cleaning. Brax walked with Lotus and said, "Okay, I'm heading to the kitchen."

"Good luck meeting with the new workers," Lotus replied.

As he walked to the back, he saw the rear door open and Master Dakor talking to two men he assumed to be the new workers. He tried to get close enough to listen but could not make out what was being said so he got even closer. At that moment, Master Dakor put his head up as if he felt Brax, then looked to the left and stared right at him.

Acting as if he had just arrived, Brax quickly asked "Are these the new employees?" Brax looked at Subdo, pretending not to recognize him.

"Yes, this is Subdo and Dred," said Master Dakor. "They will be working here."

Brax said hello. They just nodded their heads. Then Master Dakor said to Subdo and Dred, "For today, go to the grain bins. Fill five sacks of grain, deliver it to the list of orders I will give you and collect payment. Brax, you stay here and continue your work."

"Okay, sir," Brax answered, curious about where all the grain was going. When he delivered for Lotus a few days earlier, she said they never collect payment upon delivery because it was always prepaid or other arrangements were made. Many who bought the grain were local shop owners with standing agreements with her father, Master Blade.

As Brax walked into the kitchen, Master Dakor said to Subdo and Dred, "I have changed my mind. I will come with you to show you the shops."

Jade Chi Do

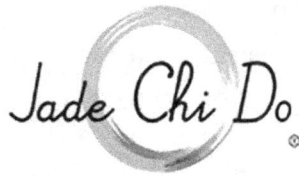

PART II - CHAPTER 6

The Discovery

Brax watched them leave with the sacks of grain, then walked out to the dining room to sweep. Thinking about what had just taken place, he almost walked into Lotus.

"Are you okay? You seem distracted," she asked.

"Yes. It's just that - it's so strange."

"What do you mean?"

"Master Dakor is going with the new hires to deliver five bags of grain. He told them before that he was going, and that they were going to collect money for the bags being delivered."

"Brax, that is not normal."

"I know."

"I have an idea," Lotus said. "Would you follow them and see what they're up to? I'll cover for you here. When you return, you can catch up with anything I didn't get to. Do you think you can do that without being noticed?"

"Okay, I must hurry then."

Brax left the Cat's Claw quickly, thinking he must apply Master Talon's lesson. He was nervous because he knew this would test the level of development of his current training. Should it not be strong enough, Master Dakor would find out. As he went down the path by the shops in the village, he saw Master Dakor walking into one of them with his new hires. Brax reminded himself that he could not give conscious attention to them, especially Master Dakor. He practiced his mirror focus and conveyed his intentions to his inner self to complete his activity. He noticed he was able to see more around him then he expected. It was a kind of hyper-awareness. He also noticed that time had no feeling. Until he had to maintain this exercise continually while following Master Dakor, he never realized how much his mind floated around.

He walked right up to the side window of the shop and listened. They did not feel him. He heard the shop owner say, "Why must I pay you?" It was hard to maintain his mirror focus and listen at first so he applied no conscious thought to it. Then he heard Master Dakor answer, "It is for your protection. If you don't pay, your family may get hurt tomorrow. But if you pay, we will protect you."

Brax heard a woman scream. He assumed it was the shopkeeper's wife. Then Master Dakor yelled, "Stop, Dred! Let her go!" He then said to the shopkeeper. "See? I can protect you."

With a frightened voice, the shopkeeper said, "Okay!"

Witnessing this, Brax became angry, disrupting his conscious mind and causing his focus to shift for only a split second. He quickly noticed the same feeling of pressure he had felt when he first met Master Dakor. Just as this happened, Master Dakor shouted, "I feel someone observing me!"

Just then, a bird flew into the shop through the open door. Startled, and her nerves on edge because of the harassment by Dakor's henchman, the shopkeeper's wife screamed and jumped back, knocking a vase off of a table. It shattered on the floor and distracted Master Dakor just long enough for Brax to reapply his special exercise. He decided he had learned enough and ran back to the Cat's Claw restaurant. Lotus saw him walk in the front door and move quickly to the kitchen. She followed him.

"Brax, are you okay? Did you find out what they're doing?"

"Yes, but let me tell you on the walk home."

Lotus went back to work not knowing why Brax was so short with her. She was very curious to find out what he had discovered, but Brax was concerned about Master Dakor coming back and figuring out it was he who had been watching him. He quickly started doing the dishes that had backed up while he was gone. He didn't see Master Dakor come back.

At the end of the evening, Brax met Lotus to walk her home. It was a bright night with many stars.

"Brax, what did you learn when you followed my uncle?" she asked.

"I saw that he loves to feed off the fear of those he intimidates. He sells a bag of grain for much more than it is worth, and he makes people pay him for protection from getting hurt."

"Protection? What do you mean by protection? From whom?"

"From him! And from the new hires."

"This makes no sense," said Lotus.

"It's extortion."

"Do you think this is the only thing he's up to?" Lotus asked.

"No. I think he's going to engage in more intimidation by finding and using the great value of this emerald to do the same thing but on a larger scale. We will continue to observe and see what else he's up to."

"My uncle did say he was hiring more workers. I told him we don't have the money to hire more than we need. He said I shouldn't worry because he was coming into some money. He was probably referring to the emerald. It sounds like he's building a gang."

"I think you're right," Brax replied. "Can you imagine him using the emerald? He could have an army."

They both became very quiet and walked a bit.

"I hope we can stop this somehow," said Lotus.

"We have cast a net. Let's observe and see where the best path that opens up to us is. There is so much we still don't know."

Trying to change the subject and lighten the mood, Brax looked up and said, "The stars sure are pretty tonight."

As Lotus looked up, a falling star raced across the sky.

"Did you see that, Brax?" she asked. She grabbed his hand, pulled him gently, and pointed to the sky.

"Yes, I was looking somewhere else, but I caught a quick glimpse of it."

"I'll make a wish," said Lotus.

Brax smiled and noticed she was still holding his hand. As he looked down at her hand, she noticed what she was doing and let go. Lotus blushed a little. Brax smiled and she gave him a little smile in return. As they passed the pond, Brax remembered how her

reflection glowed that night.

"I enjoyed skipping rocks with you in the moonlight the other night," said Brax.

"You told me that before," she said, giggling.

"Oh, yeah."

"But it's okay. I enjoyed it too. My father has shared so much with me, and some real cool stuff by this pond."

"Your father loves you very much."

"Yes, he is such a wise person."

When they reached Lotus's house, she said, "Let's hope tomorrow is a better day."

"It will be - the moment I see you smile," Brax said, surprised that he let himself say that. It just kind of popped out.

"You have such a great outlook," said Lotus. She felt a rush of warmth come over her.

"Goodnight, Lotus."

She smiled and went inside. As he was walking home, he reviewed how his training had saved him, and also what he felt when he had allowed himself to be distracted. When he arrived, he looked forward to hearing what Master Talon would say when he told him what had happened.

The next morning, Brax walked to the shop for his morning lesson as Master Talon had instructed him to do. This time, as he got close to the pond, he immediately saw Master Talon sitting in the chair by the tree next to the path. He stopped in front of him.

"How was your day yesterday?" Master Talon asked.

"You were right, unfortunately. Master Dakor feeds on this fear energy frequency. He is very sensitive. I slipped up for a few seconds and let my conscious mind get angry. It distracted me from the exercise, which was working wonderfully until I did that. He felt my presence immediately."

"Brax, you will learn more as you become more sensitive to yourself. Anger is very powerful, even though it sends energy everywhere, especially when not focused. It's like a fire alarm bell - it radiates outward."

"He seems to be building a gang, or worse - a large army of bandits. Why do you think he's doing this?"

Master Talon grew very serious. "The trouble with projecting and feeding from the cold force is that it gives into fear, which creates a hunger of sorts that compels them to seek power outside of themselves. This explains his desire to acquire power this way. Also, to defeat those that challenge him, he knows he must form a group of impressionable men under his influence. Let's walk over to the same tree in the field across from this path. It is time for your next lesson. Do you remember the previous lesson's exercise we did there?"

"Yes. Very well."

"Good."

When they arrived at the tree, Master Talon said, "Our goal here today is to work on sensitivity within yourself. We must train so that this field of energy within your warm life force becomes its own definition. That way, your personal blinders cannot hide what was there all along. By being aware of this, it will be as tangible as touching an apple and being able to taste it. You can then either hold the apple or throw it. Think of it this way - before you knew what an orange was, you first had to eat it and taste it. Soon afterward, it became its own definition. If you were blind and had only eaten oranges your whole life, then were given a green apple to bite, would you not say that that was a very hard and sour orange? That is, until you were taught that it was an apple? Do you understand?"

"Yes, I do."

"Now review what I just said about the apple and replace the word apple with this energy of our *warm life force* we speak about," said Master Talon.

"I have never thought of it that way. Seeing it like that will definitely help my mind stay open. I see even more now the importance of your teaching through explanation, not just showing me moves," said Brax.

"We are going deeper into your training because your task with Master Dakor gives me no choice but to accelerate you. Be sure that your choice is focused on the warm force. When one is accelerated without years of training, the discipline of making the right choice can be more difficult. This is also why I'm teaching you this way right now. You have already mastered several fighting arts. We are in the next level of your training. Your prior arts were like being given a gun. What I am teaching you is the part from within that pulls the trigger."

"Thank you, Master. I see that you are opening my perspective so I am more able to learn and achieve what you're teaching me. If I understand you correctly, you are teaching me to discover that which is already within me."

Always the type of student looking to advance to the next level, Brax added, "How may I increase the effectiveness of my training?"

"Those who are able to extend their view beyond their own ego - that is, how great they see themselves - will learn and achieve much," said Master Talon. "The next step of today's lesson starts now."

Jade Chi Do

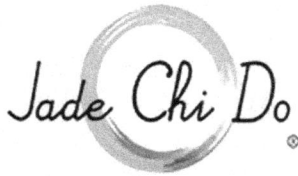

PART II - CHAPTER 7

Questions

Master Talon looked at Brax for a minute and said, "Let's sit here in the field. We need to talk some more." After they both sat down, he continued, "Brax, because of your impending conflict with Master Dakor, it is good that you have already mastered your previous martial styles. What I am teaching you now accesses that which is already within you, and much more. To fully access and move this warm life force, you must be aware of it tangibly. Today's lesson will be your stepping stone."

Brax replied, "Master, if I may ask, are you ever concerned that some whom you teach will not be able or willing to access your lessons?"

"This is possible. I screen and test potential students, but I have learned that those who do not learn in the way I teach are simply not ready to hear it so it may make no sense to them. Or, due to ego or pride, they write it off as something they have learned elsewhere and miss out on what is really being taught. This causes loss to its tangible achievements. Therefore, I have less concern for how much of what I teach is received than I did when I was younger."

"Master Talon, why is Master Dakor so much younger than you? It doesn't make sense based on what you told me about your past together."

"When Master Dakor came to my teacher as a very young man, he had tremendous natural sensitivity. Because there were only three of us, our teacher became very fond of us. My teacher said it was our duty to share what we had learned with those who were ready to see, and who wanted to accomplish more than they were able to. We did so, and these people became much better at what they did in their lives. When they reached mastery, they were also given the parting task of sharing this with others who were ready. But enough of this for now. As you know, the purpose of this lesson is not to teach you combat. I am accelerating your training to amplify your access to the warm force within you. Now let's work on removing your blinders so there will be no restrictions left. This training will allow you to access this force and react in times of need with much greater effect - whether in life, art, or whatever profession you choose. Its immediate purpose is to prepare you for the conflict with Master Dakor. I know you can defend yourself, but in the coming situation, you will need to access a deeper connection within yourself and be aware of your higher abilities. You may have had small glances of them, moments when you've felt hints of their greatness within you. You are already a master of a few styles. Now it is time for the next level."

"Is this why I have seen so many businessmen, professional athletes, and martial art masters come to your shop?" asked Brax.

"Yes. This next step will help you shake off the blinders you have - that all people unknowingly attach to themselves. But to increase your life's accomplishments, you must be willing to go further than others are willing or able to - and most of the time, it's *able*, not *willing*, because very few know what I am about to teach you."

"I can already see how this would help anyone in business or sports that require a heightened skill level," said Brax.

"Good, then it is time to begin," said Master Talon.

They both stood up, then Master Talon said, "Stand twenty paces from the tree. Today, you are not going to look at it as a mirror of the tree; just look at it and relate to it. A tree does not think as we do. It does not feel the wind that touched it yesterday, or even a second ago, nor does it feel the wind tomorrow or even a second ahead of the present moment. So look at the tree in this new way. Do not provide conscious thought to it. Relate to it in your mind. See it feeling the wind at the same moment you do, with no thought."

After allowing Brax some time to accomplish this, the master added, "Now we're going to do the first exercise of Heaven and Earth. To recap a little, stand with your arms on your side with your feet shoulder-width apart. Breathe and do the exercise as I previously taught you. Apply a deeper attention, moving with very slow motion. At the same time, see your breath pulling and pushing through the body, connecting to your breath, moving inward on your inhale and outward on your exhale. You should root first without bending your knees. Do this three times. When you finish, start bending your knees on the inhale. On the exhale, begin to straighten your legs as you visualize your breath with warm life force, seeing the flow go out through your hands and feet. Do the opposite on the inhale."

Master Talon again observed as Brax finished the exercise. When he was done, he said, "Now we will awaken and discover that which has been waiting within you. The third time, as your hands drop toward your sides, instead of your palms moving toward your legs, move them forward in front of you just enough so that both hands are facing each other slightly but are still facing forward. Do this on the third repeat of the duplicate movement, in this first part of the exercise. Start it on the exhale. Continue repeating the first part of the Heaven and Earth exercise that I have taught you. Next, alternate the regular exercise and the new exercise. Between the two of them, pay attention to any difference you feel from your palms, and from within your body. You will start to feel something that your blinders have been hiding from you. Do not be excited or alarmed or it will fade. Do not try to define it. Just exist in the exercise. Go back to doing the regular exercise two times, then on the third time, do the new exercise. Continue to visualize."

Brax practiced this exercise, adding the extra moves on the third part. He felt an amazing pressure, yet it really was not pressure. He became a little confused and asked, "Master Talon, what is this feeling? At first, I thought it was pressure, but it's really more like a kind of warmth, even though my hands aren't hot."

Master Talon laughed happily. "Now I know you are on the right path. This will soon become its own defined feeling. Remember our talk a little bit ago about the apple? It is like you are calling the green apple a sour orange. It is time to discover the apple. If I am going to teach you how to throw or move the apple, you first must definitely know it is an apple to do so fully. Many on the path of discovering this new sense realize that it was always there. Our body tries to define it in terms we already know, like warm, cold, hot, pressure, tingling, and many other sense files we have, until it finally becomes its own file; it's own sense. No longer will it be hidden by your blinders. Thereafter, one can feel and recognize it in others and its use can be grown much faster."

Brax practiced this for most of his training time. When he was done, Master Talon said, "Brax before you leave today, I have one more lesson for you to practice. Do this same exercise with your eyes closed. There are two main changes - visualize seeing yourself doing the movements as if you are the mirror watching or observing yourself. At the same time, your conscious focus is on the moment of the exercise. Here is where it gets tricky: just as a tree seeks to align with gravity, allow yourself to be aware of your body aligning with this. You will feel any tipping or movement more with your eyes closed while you're standing doing the exercises. When you do the third new exercise, you will feel a heightened sensitivity to this warm life force you called a feeling of pressure with warmth. In reality, you are discovering and creating its new file because it was always already there."

"How do I discover and create? It is one or the other, isn't it?" asked Brax.

"Brax, have you ever picked an apple off a tree?" asked Master Talon.

"Yes."

"Was the apple always there?"

"Yes."

"Could you see the apple from your home, far away?"

"No."

"Of course not. First, you would need to walk up to the tree, then look up to see the apple. Would you say you discovered it?"

"Yes, if I did not see it before."

"What then must you do to get the apple?"

"I must reach up to grab the apple," Brax replied.

"So you choose to create a path to grab the apple?"

"Yes. I see what you mean. I know this is just a basic explanation, but I understand the deeper message you are giving me," said Brax.

"This is good! You are finding what I was trying to say to you instead of trying to poke holes in it. When a student tries to finds holes in a lesson, it is just their blinders trying to keep their minds closed and in a limited paradigm."

"Why do people resist change?" Brax asked.

"Growth of any kind usually involves emotions that are uncomfortable, such as confusion. A wise student bound for great things understands that confusion is only a doorway to higher understanding and awareness, and embraces this stage of learning by staying aware of what is on the other side of it. There's an old saying - if you do what others won't for a year, you'll have what they can't for the rest of your life. Do you understand?"

"Yes," Brax replied.

"Another reason people resist growth and try to discredit new information is self-sabotage, or fearing reaching a higher level and becoming someone else. But their fundamental self and nature doesn't change; they simply become a better, higher version of themselves - the person they were always meant to be. In turn, though friends and others may be jealous of their abilities at first, they become an inspiration to them later, as those who walk through the fire of their own doubts and fears always are."

Inspired by this new insight, Brax returned to his practice and was amazed by what he felt. Noticing his progress, Master Talon asked, "What do you feel as you do the exercise and get to the new third part?"

"While feeling the alignment, I felt a little trance, like being in a zone of its own. I did feel three points of a sort of momentary oneness.

I felt that warm pressure I told you about in my hands. The difference was that I felt this not only in my palms but also in my head - almost between my eyes, I think."

"Good! Through practice, this path will increase your sense of this force and a new sense file will soon emerge," said Master Talon. "As a tree seeks to align with this invisible force of gravity, so we also align with it in this exercise. Practice the awareness of this feeling as you walk. Walking to work will be a good time for this. But as I taught you earlier, do not stop being aware of all your vision around you. Remember, just because we can't see gravity doesn't mean it doesn't exist. This warm life force exists in the same way."

"I have another question," Brax said. "Will this undo any of my styles I have learned?"

"No, it won't. I know you don't want to lose any techniques you've learned because you will need them for the future conflict with Master Dakor. You still must maintain your physical training. This training is not competitive, it's complementary. It will enhance and amplify what you already know. To receive massive results from what I teach you, you must know this difference very deeply within yourself, with a high level of confidence."

"Is this taught in the same way as my other arts?" asked Brax.

"Yes, just as many styles, methods and arts teach techniques that use small resistance training, which builds the body up to a higher tolerance of that resistance. In many cases, the body's health increases. We practice this from within ourselves, connecting to outwardly exercises. With properly taught techniques, the body will adapt, like slowly introducing cold or other factors. Your body can counteract many kinds of harm. It will increase health in many respects by building up resistance to threats to the body. Here's a less complex example - your hand acquires calluses for protection. If resistance is done too quickly and not over time, it will become a blister before it has time to build into calluses. So whether it be over cold or any threat to the body, from holding one's breath to breaking a brick, with proper teaching, one can achieve much more. I am not teaching you a physical resistance style like these. I hope this explains your concern."

Brax nodded. "I see now. Jade Chi Do will sharpen the sword - that is, my style I already have within me. I will also begin to notice the abilities I have earned in those other styles begin to grow stronger."

"Very good. This is why I have moved your training to Jade Chi Do," said Master Talon. "As the sensitivity to the warm force grows, it will shine and demonstrate itself in all that you do, including your arts, business, sports, and more. Use of this warm life force can only accelerate what you are trained in, no different than you mastering your other martial art styles. This special art of Jade Chi Do is an accelerated complement to any of these styles."

"Master Talon, you said to me that the warm force is life and it is always moving, from a human cell to a walking person. What do you mean?" Brax asked.

"Let me ask you a question, Brax. If you were walking toward a destination and you fell down, what would you do?"

"I would stand up."

"Why?"

"Because if I just stayed down, I would never get to where I was going."

"What if you laid there for a long time, not moving?"

"I would eventually die."

"Would you say, then, that to move is life?"

"Yes."

"Do you get warm if you walk or exercise for a while?"

"Yes."

"Would you say that this is life as well?"

"Yes."

"Then to use your life force chi in a stronger way, what would you add to your current static meditations?"

Brax thought for a moment when the realization hit him; the proverbial light bulb turning on. He smiled, excited.

"Motion! I learn through Jade Chi Do!"

"Yes. Jade Chi Do teaches inner motion that is not seen while simultaneously connecting to the forces of our outer motion," Master

Talon said. "The body then rewards us as we interact with life, and we discover we have more capabilities than we had previously perceived."

Brax looked up at the sun and saw that it was getting late. The time had flown quickly.

"I must go to work now, Master Talon. I will practice," said Brax.

"Remember, as you walk, maintain focus, yet see all around yourself. Your exercise today will reflect out of you in an amazing way. Now go," said Master Talon.

Brax left, reviewing his lesson as he walked along. Seeing this taught with an exercise gave him perspective to better absorb the techniques. As he walked down the path, he started to practice what Master Talon instructed.

Jade Chi Do

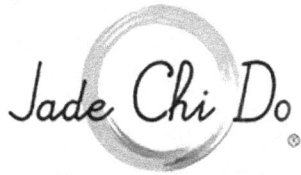

PART II - CHAPTER 8

The Challenge

Brax began to notice that he was viewing things a little differently without even trying. Oddly, he often felt as if he were looking out of a wide windscreen in a carriage and he was the driver. He saw more than he expected. He noticed what he had just gone over with Master Talon as he practiced. He first started walking a little slower to get a feel for the gravity he was aligning himself with. He made his strides more timed and coordinated. As he did, he began to have a feeling of tipping back-and-forth and side-to-side, becoming more sensitive to the pull of gravity as he walked.

Then he added the other exercise given to him by Master Talon. As he walked and looked ahead, he applied little conscious thought, although he was fully aware. He observed the center of the path and his peripheral vision simultaneously. As Master Talon predicted, he was able to see all around himself while maintaining a general focus on a spot at the center of the path before him. For a second or two, things seemed to go in slow motion, but as soon as he noticed it and gave it conscious attention, it vanished.

As he continued to walk, a rabbit ran across the path about thirty paces in front of him. When he was in the depth of practicing, as he watched the rabbit, it seemed to be running in slow motion. Realizing this ability was growing in him made him feel excited. This filled his mind with conscious thought, which made the rabbit return to normal speed like a slingshot in his mind. He tried to recreate this event but was too excited and full of questions. He tried again and again but was not able to do it.

As he approached the Cat's Claw, he noticed a group of people standing in front of the restaurant. He walked by them and entered the front door to ask Lotus what was happening. She saw Brax arrive, came over to him and excitedly said good morning.

Brax felt a rush of warmth in his stomach as he looked into her eyes.

"It has just begun to be a good morning, now that I'm seeing you."

"Yeah, like I am the sunshine," Lotus responded. She laughed shyly, flattered and surprised by his kind words.

"What's with the crowd out there?" asked Brax. "I don't know,"

Lotus replied.

They both heard a loud, gong-like sound from outside and looked out the window.

"Look! It's Master Dakor practicing sparring with his men," Lotus said. They both walked outside. Brax immediately thought this must be a show of force by Master Dakor to intimidate his present and future victims. Brax looked at Dred as he shouted out to the crowd.

"Want to win this big bag of coins?" Dred yelled, raising the bag above his shoulders as he spoke. "All you have to do is join in a friendly sparring match with Master Dakor. To win, you must not fall to the ground before the last grain of sand falls in this hourglass." The hourglass had about five minute's worth of sand and sat on a table next to where Master Dakor was standing. Master Dakor announced to the crowd, which was mostly made up of shopkeepers, that he would not seriously hurt anyone.

A few of the heartier men tried their luck but no one could last five minutes with him. Brax thought it strange that Master Dakor somehow put fear in them, though he couldn't see how. Each came on strong but seemed to quickly lose their drive and strength, then concede before the five minutes was up. Master Dakor looked over to Brax with a deep grin and said to the crowd, "Now this young man has the courage to win this prize! Come on over, Brax."

Brax felt out of place. He immediately thought that if he won, he would put the extra money away to return to the shop owners. Then he thought *The net is cast. I do not want to bring attention to this.*

"You don't have to do this, Brax," Lotus said, with worry in her voice. Brax felt like Lotus thought he would fail. That's when his pride got the better of him and he blurted out, "I accept!" He knew he was a good martial artist and could last five minutes easily. He planned to just focus and not let Master Dakor break down his confidence as he had been doing to everyone else.

The hourglass was flipped and the time started. They circled and Master Dakor seemed to push himself into Brax mentally until he couldn't think straight. He bested Brax several times. Brax's ego disrupted his focus again as he feared looking bad in front of Lotus. Master Dakor knew this and said to the crowd, "The young man is weak!"

This made Brax rush one of his favorite techniques on Master Dakor, one that always worked against his fellow students, but it had no effect on Master Dakor. It was as if he knew what he was going to do ahead of time. He just slapped Brax lightly on the chest. The slap felt like a cold vibration going through him. His energy left him, as if his quick burst of anger had pulled the strength out of him. He fell to the ground for a few seconds just as the last bit of sand slipped through the hourglass and his time was up. He stood as Master Dakor spoke to the crowd, instilling more fear in them, "Even this young man could not last!"

Lotus grabbed Brax's hand and pulled him away. "I want you to take a full day off tomorrow," she said.

"I'm okay. I don't need a day off," said Brax.

"Trust me," Lotus implored. "My father has taught me there is a time for this. It recharges one's outlook."

Brax conceded, but his ego was a little bruised.

"We can meet two days from now and go fish in the pond," said Lotus.

They both finished the day at the restaurant. Brax walked Lotus home without speaking much. She could tell he had a lot on his mind.

"Do you suspect Master Dakor thinks we are trying to find out what he's doing?" asked Lotus.

"No, I didn't feel that from him, but I did feel he was trying to intimidate the shopkeepers, and used me to do so," said Brax, still a little discouraged, and angry that he allowed Master Dakor to distract and overpower him.

"A day off will help you, Brax," said Lotus.

They arrived at Lotus' house and Brax said goodnight. She looked at him and said, "My father shared a saying with me - 'If a runner runs a race, he still must rest to be the best.' Brax, I know you're the best. See you tomorrow after work. Goodnight."

This cheered Brax up. They both parted with warm smiles.

When he got home, he reflected on the day. He looked forward to having a full day of training with Master Talon the next day.

As he walked down the path to Master Talon's shop the next morning, he looked forward to training all day. All he had on his schedule was walking Lotus home after she got off work, which he also looked forward to. His pride was still hurt from sparring with Master Dakor and looked forward to going over this with Master Talon.

When he arrived, Master Talon was in front of the shop.

"Good morning," said Brax.

Master Talon observed him for a moment and said, "Good morning. What's wrong? I feel that you're a little distressed."

Brax was surprised because he didn't think he had revealed anything to Master Talon, but he had learned not to question his abilities.

"I'm shaken by a sparring match I had with Master Dakor. He was putting on an exhibition for a crowd in front of the restaurant and got me to spar with him. I wasn't able to match him. It was embarrassing because I feel Lotus may not see me as proficient as I know I am. He had a way of getting into my head and pulling triggers. Anyway, what are we working on today?"

"Let's start on your perception," said Master Talon. "In any conflict, one's perception is heightened through practice so much, to watch and to react almost become one. There is a higher conscious thought and a lower conscious thought. The further you are from any lower conscious thought, the faster your reaction time is. When this is performed well, you will find that if a person were watching, they would assume that you were perceiving the action before it was coming. They would also see you giving a proper reaction. The key, of course, is to give the *right* reaction. This is based on the training you engaged in prior to Jade Chi Do. Your prior training is the toolbox you give yourself, like a mechanic. A mechanic has a motor to work on; you have a fight. A mechanic needs to find the right tool to turn the right bolt, and you need to access your tools. With dedicated Jade Chi Do training, you will effectively see what is coming and interact with it accordingly. You become simply a watcher, seeing it at its inception before it happens. But without prior tools and actions to draw from, you will just see it instead of yourself effectively reacting. That said, there are many who are able to react properly to situations from somewhere deep within with less training."

"Master Talon," Brax said, "with my further training, will I learn a special way to interpret what I see and react to?"

"Brax, we are the same and different and unique to ourselves all at the same time, meaning your path to seeing what is coming may be different from another's path in some ways, yet still achieve the same thing - seeing it. But one's style - or tools - to react to it also comes into effect. For example, I see trails where another sees it played out milliseconds before it arises."

Master Talon thought for a moment, then continued, "Here's another good example. I had a great student. He was a master of his style. After he completed his sessions with me, he said a type of light showed him the direction of the attack. He then saw himself reacting to this like a dance. He even said that after using this, a higher thought would happen. He could think without engaging his conscious mind -

the part that thinks out loud to ourselves. I have learned that the masters I train create a unique pathway of communication from their conscious mind to their higher selves."

"Okay," Brax said, "so If I understand this properly, whatever skills or styles I have learned become my tools for my actions and reactions to access?"

"Yes. But this awareness can translate to business, sports, and many activities. Being more connected to your body as a whole source increases the health of the mind as well as the body. It is very important for you to know that you don't need to learn a different style first to study Jade Chi Do. It is helpful, but if you practice Jade Chi Do then learn a new style, sport, or profession, when you need to react quickly to a situation, it will serve you well. You will find that you will learn and assimilate it much deeper and faster."

"How may I make this process happen faster for me?" asked Brax. "When Master Dakor invited me to spar with him, my pride thought - actually, it was more like a command - that I should show him my great skill, so I did, but he seemed to read every movement before I did them. Due to my Jade Chi Do training so far, I recognized and felt his cold force feeding on me, drawing out my uncertainty. This made me feel unbalanced."

"He is trying to control you by instilling fear. The cold force is his tool," said Master Talon. "Many unknowingly use this, as I mentioned before. It is not evil or good, but one should not feed this action because the use of it is destructive to oneself. A technique of basic fighters and bar brawlers is to come on very powerfully by sending out vibrations of massive action and anger. The cold force cuts into the opponent and tips the scale many times to win the fight, especially to the untrained. These unscrupulous people continue to intensify the fear in others well past its original perceived use. This power becomes intoxicating, and those who choose to continue this intensity seek it like food. But like all hungers, the need to replenish the fuel source is endless. Sadly, it is outside themselves, and it comes at a cost to others. There is a place in war for this but the overwhelming force given to the trained will identify this and offer two choices - to react at its inception when it is easier to detour or direct its force before momentum starts - or to fight fire with fire. But with that approach, much energy is lost and the battle of longevity starts to find its victor. This is the usual strategy in cage fighting, but where there are multiple attackers, fire against fire makes one bigger fire. Another may come from the sidelines with water and be the victor."

"How did he do this to me?" asked Brax.

"No matter how good you are, if one intrudes on you internally, this can happen. Further training is needed for you to project the use of your own warm force."

How may I increase the effectiveness of Jade Chi Do?" asked Brax.

"Like anything else, to build success - be it muscle memory or a talent or profession - we must demonstrate to ourselves that it is important to us. To build a smooth communication for this starts with one word - repetition; in our case, visual repetition as well. Any martial art, be it regular or a mixture, is indeed all mixed anyway. It is all tools you grab from your toolbox to react to the situation. I am here to help with the reaction time - that is, the space in which the watcher sees. Now, like a hand building a callus, let's increase some friction to your inner self to find out if this is what you really want."

Jade Chi Do

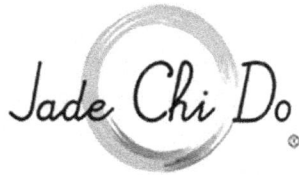

PART II - CHAPTER 9

To See Without Seeing

"**B**rax, before we go inside, pick up three stones about the size of your palm," said Master Talon.

Brax looked around the front area of the shop and found three round, golf ball-size stones. Master Talon saw this and said, "Follow me."

They both walked through the shop toward the back area where Brax usually trained. When they reached the door, Master Talon stopped him before he could exit.

"Brax, give me the stones, please."

Brax handed him the stones and Master Talon walked over to the table where they usually have tea. He placed the rocks in line on the table, about a hand or so apart from each other, in front of where Brax normally sits.

"As you come through the doorway, look at the three rocks as you walk toward them. Before you get to the table, turn and sit on the bench seat, in front of the rocks. Then sit facing the doorway through which you entered. Without looking, reach around and grab the middle rock. Touch no other rock. You will need to continue imagining and remembering, as if you're still looking at the rocks. The purpose of the exercise is to see - that is, visualize - your hand going around your body and grabbing the rock with precision, as if you were seeing it with your own eyes."

Brax did so but brushed against the wrong rock on his first try. Master Talon saw that he was getting a little frustrated.

"Brax, this is why we are practicing this now. Visual repetition is key."

"I thought this was going to be just like shadow boxing. I was so wrong," Brax said.

"I see. Even though you did not want to interpret this lesson based on another style, you did," said Master Talon.

"Yes."

"I did the same thing many times," Master Talon said. "My teacher said I needed to stop racing ahead of what was being taught because I was assuming what the lesson was rather than recognizing it as new information. Therefore, I was missing the deeper meaning of lessons, not learning anything new, only what I assumed. In other words, I was recycling information I already possessed, not accepting new knowledge. My ego was filling in the teaching too soon by assuming instead of really listening. How, then, could I say the art was not working? We must recognize every moment as unique, without diluting it through comparison, and not just in Jade Chi Do but in all things. We can savor and enjoy every moment, or compare and dilute them to past events and old knowledge. Again, to truly achieve the benefits, one must catch oneself when this happens. If not, the fruits of Jade Chi Do cannot help you, and the cold force will feed on your ego. It will be hard to learn more than you already know. If we stop learning, where does this leave us but in disorder - a prime deceptive goal of the cold force."

Brax thought about this for a few moments, then said, "Master Talon, I have noticed when I watch sports that some of what you call the cold force is used to intimidate the other team's players."

Master Talon nodded and said, "If one uses the cold force of intimidation in a game, he must give much time to the warm force. If not, he will be prone to much anger, and the lasting effects will not just be unhealthy, but very destructive.

When Brax had time to digest this information, Master Talon continued, "I want you to start the exercise again. Use your whole vision from our previous training. Do not have much conscious thought but know and communicate your goals to your inner self by seeing what is required."

Brax went to the doorway and reflected for a moment on what Master Talon said about his interpretation of some of his lessons. At first, he felt his ego defend himself, but then he laughed when he recognized this and said to himself, "I'm going to learn more than what I think I know." The moment he said this, Master Talon felt a sort of light appear and shine from within Brax. He immediately said, "Start your practice now."

Brax did, and this time he didn't touch any other rock, only the middle one. Master Talon instructed, "Continue to do the exercise, alternating the rocks you pick up until I tell you to stop,"

Brax performed this exercise many times until he got very good at it. Master Talon noticed this and said, "Now go stand by the doorway again. Let me move a few of the rocks." He then moved them all around the table in different locations. They repeated this many times. When he was proficient at this exercise, Master Talon said, "It's time to accelerate your teaching some more. I will now walk as you watch me from the doorway. I will place the rock in different locations in this area. Walk up to it, then turn and reach around to grab it."

Master Talon placed the rocks at different heights as well. This went on for a long time as he observed Brax's progress.

"Okay, Brax. One last exercise for today. Go to the doorway and face me again. I will put the three rocks back on the table."

Master Talon walked over to Brax, handed him a blindfold and had him put it on. When he did, Master Talon walked back to the table and said, "Pull your blindfold up enough to see where I placed the rocks on the table. Don't try to memorize this but keep the active picture of what you see in the way we were just training. Then lower the blindfold, walk over, and grab the middle rock." Brax did so, and to his amazement, he grabbed the middle rock.

They practiced this many times. Next, they did the same exercise they had done without the blindfold earlier in the day. Master Talon placed one rock. Brax watched before he pulled the blindfold down. Brax navigated around the obstacles and picked the rock up.

To surprise Brax, Master Talon told him to walk back without taking his blindfold off. Brax had a second of nervousness that nearly blinded him from the picture he was seeing. He calmed himself, and as he turned to face the doorway, he visualized a picture. It appeared from his inner self, and he was able to see the path he needed to walk to return to the doorway. He did so without error. Brax was amazed.

Master Talon said, "Next, look at me and place one rock on the table. After you lower the blindfold, I will move the rock to a different spot on this same table. I will do some projection of myself in this action, which will help you accelerate this. Now let's begin."

"How do I do this?" asked Brax.

"Look for the pressure or warm feeling you said you felt. It's the sense of the warm force that will guide you. You will feel a subtle feeling - a magnetic kind of pull or push."

Brax was a little nervous because he thought this was just a memory exercise - and this went beyond memory. Again, he caught himself assuming. He then started the exercise. He looked, then lowered the blindfold, and began to walk over. As he got close, he went to grab the rock. Just as his right hand got close to the spot on the table where he last saw it, he felt a warm tingle in his thumb. It was very faint, then there was a sort of pull to the left, like weak gravity pulling on him, or a swinging pendulum. Brax followed it as his hand dropped more. He then felt a sort of mixture of feelings, like hot and cold at the same time. He then grabbed the rock. Just as Brax was going to cheer in amazement, Master Talon said, "Stop. Now, to help increase your sensitivity to this, I will need you to place the rock in my hand. Extend it outward. I will amplify my attention to receiving it. You may feel this."

Master Talon was testing Brax. If he had confidence in his training and had practiced with an empty cup, he would indeed set the rock in Master Talon's hands. Brax turned toward his voice and lifted the rock up a little higher in front of himself. He felt Master Talon's presence as he reached out. He felt the hand as if he was watching from a mirror. He then dropped the rock in Master Talon's palm.

When he didn't hear the rock hit the floor, Brax opened his eyes and saw Master Talon holding the rock and smiling. Brax was curious about how and where this training would show itself, knowing that all Master Talon's training exercises were like a recipe leading to something much greater. This showed him he was on the right track.

"Today's exercise is done," said Master Talon. "Let's sit and reflect a bit, and have some tea before you go home."

As they sat drinking tea, Brax asked, "How was it that I saw a picture, like watching a mirror, that allowed me to see where to place the rock in your hand?"

Master Talon replied, "Each student's inner self may communicate this information differently, while having the same outcome. It was a test to see how well integrated and connected the sum of the cumulative achievements from your previous training is. In other words, your self was accessing all your training. I, as the teacher, was seeing how you had integrated it together to achieve greater use of the warm force. It is not just physical or not physical; it is the unity of a combined action. Basically, this means you are digesting and your blinders are slowly being lifted. If you practice right, focusing on the training - the recipe - you will find that it takes much less conscious effort than you have previously imagined. It is the responsibility of the teacher to install this in a way that brings the least amount of resistance from the student's unique blinders. The quality of practice accelerates a student's learning. Brax, you may be surprised how today's training will integrate into your life. This will help you in your pending conflict with Master Dakor."

Brax asked, "May I ask why I felt two impossible feelings at the same time? It doesn't make sense how I felt it as a cold and hot feeling simultaneously."

Master Talon smiled very warmly and said, "My dear Brax, this is a sign that you are getting close to that apple becoming its own definition and feeling. Soon your blinders will no longer be able to blind you to this."

Brax felt a little more enlightened but still full of questions. He knew that he would learn more soon. He said, "Thank you for your time. It feels so good to have a full day of talk and instruction with you." He gave Master Talon a kernel of corn from the cob, as he had instructed him to do after each day's lesson when he first started training months earlier, but Master Talon politely refused it.

"Not now, Brax. We can resume this when your normal training starts again; when this is all over. Do not lose it, for it is a lesson in itself."

Brax agreed and said, "I must leave now to walk Lotus home."

"Practice and reflect on your lessons," Master Talon said. "And be careful, Brax.

Jade Chi Do

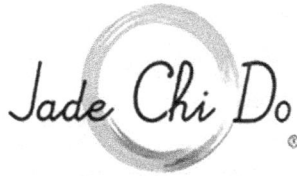

PART II - CHAPTER 10

New Beginnings

L otus was coming out of the restaurant as Brax arrived. They exchanged greetings and started walking home. Lotus was very quiet, thinking deeply about something. For a moment, Brax thought he could spend the rest of his life just walking with her and never be bored for a moment. He enjoyed the silence at first because he knew that one of the best ways to know when two people have become very close is when silence ceases to be uncomfortable. However, his curiosity got the better of him and he asked her what she was thinking.

"I'm trying to relax," she replied. "My father once told me, 'When you need to find an answer to a problem you're worried about, you must detach from it and wait. If not, your tension creates a dam that holds back a river of solutions from getting to you. You must let go to receive. A good sleep or a day off is helpful.' By the way, did your day off help you?"

"Yes, it did," Brax said. "At first, my mind was still stuck on the events of the day before, but when I put my full mental effort into my training, everything improved."

When they reached her doorway, she said, "I feel we will have better plans tomorrow.

They said goodnight and Brax walked home, meditating on her father's wise words.

The next morning, Brax walked into the Cat's Claw and found Lotus cleaning the front window of the dining room. They greeted each other and Lotus said, "Guess what? It came to me!"

"What came to you?" asked Brax.

"I have an idea. I have been worried about you following Master Dakor the way you have been because of that close call you told me about the other day."

"What are you thinking?"

"I suggest you ask Master Dakor for extra work so you can get paid more money. I know extra money is not your motivation, but this is a way to get closer to what's happening without having to follow him."

"Interesting," Brax said.

"Let me tell you a story," Lotus suggested. "One day, my father and I were fishing for trout and he said, 'A hook is made to look like a fly. The fish must think it's an insect or it may not propel itself into the air where it is vulnerable and lacks all of its strength and abilities.'"

"Wow! Master Blade - I mean, your father - has much wisdom," Brax said.

"Thank you. My father said he named me Lotus because the moment he looked at me, he felt a great hidden wisdom that would reflect in my life - like my name, as a Lotus rising up out of the swamp and grime of this world and opening up to become a beautiful flower."

"I can see where he got the beautiful part," said Brax, with a warm smile. Lotus blushed and smiled shyly. "I will ask Master Dakor for more work. I think you're right - this will also be good practice for my training with Master Talon."

"Does Master Dakor know he is your teacher?" asked Lotus.

"No."

"That's good. Working closely with Master Dakor will help us discover more. Let's have dinner after we close the restaurant, before we head home," said Lotus.

Brax suddenly felt little butterflies in his stomach and became warm with excitement at the thought of having dinner with Lotus.

"Okay, great!" he said. "I see Master Dakor by the grain bins. I'll go ask him now." Brax was taught to not procrastinate when he had a challenging task. He knew if he had delayed it until later, it would only play on his fears or worries and increase the possibility of being discovered.

"Be careful asking, Brax. This is still dangerous," Lotus said.

He did not reply, but gave a nod with his head. They left each other and went back to work. He walked over to Master Dakor while he was checking the level of the three grain bins, each containing different grains. He turned as Brax walked up to him.

With a firm voice and intimidating look, he said, "What do you want, Brax?"

"I need to make more money. I see you're selling more grain. Can I help deliver it for a half hour after work?"

"I have a few new hires coming on already, but they are coming from far away so they won't be starting for a couple of days. I will let you help this time. After your work, I will have Subdo get you to help carry the sacks of grain and such."

"Thank you, sir."

Brax went to wash the dishes. Lotus's grandmother asked him to take out the trash. As he walked out the rear door, he noticed a board mounted on the right side of the wall at about shoulder height. When he returned from taking out the garbage, he took a closer look at it. It was about a foot in diameter and looked like a square bamboo cutting board. As he looked closer, he saw that the board had a bolt in all four corners with springs behind it. He noticed an imprint that was a darker shade. It was in the shape of a hand. Brax was very curious about what this might be.

As he walked back into the kitchen, he saw Lotus's grandmother so he asked, "Tessa, do you know what that board is on the wall?"

"No, not exactly," she replied, "but I have heard my son Master Blade call it a 4bolt board. He places his hand on it as he bends at the knees. He then stands up a little and the board makes a snapping sound."

"Very interesting. Thank you,"

Brax went back to work. The day dragged on longer than usual because he couldn't wait to have dinner with Lotus. Every now and then, they would exchange smiles as they passed each other. The end of the day finally came. As the last customer left the dining room, Lotus's grandmother already had a dish prepared for them at the corner table. As they both walked up to sit, Tessa lit a candle on the table.

"If you two don't need anything more, I will be going home," Tessa said.

"No, we don't, Grandmother. Thank you for preparing this for us," said Lotus.

They began to eat. As Lotus was talking, Brax looked into her eyes and noticed the reflection of the flickering candle flame in them. It was almost hypnotizing to him.

"When I look into your eyes, it feels like forever could pass in a second. I could never get enough of this," he said.

Lotus was about to answer when Master Dakor's men walked in. It was the first two hires, Subdo and Dred.

"It is time," Subdo said. "Are you ready? We must go!"

Brax didn't want to leave but knew this was the plan.

"Lotus, I must leave. I'll be back in about thirty minutes."

"I'll wait here and prepare some food for tomorrow's work," Lotus replied.

Brax could hear the sad and worried tone of her voice. To calm her nerves, he said, "Okay, see you soon!" trying to sound cheerful.

"Let's go," Subdo said bluntly.

As they left to go to the back where the grain bins were, Subdo said, "We must fill eight bags of grain, four from the number one bin, two from the number two bin, and two bags of the larger grain from the number three bin." Brax had never seen anyone deliver the number three grain so far.

After they filled the grain bags, the wheelbarrow was filled with number one and number two grains. This left two bags of the larger grain.

"Brax, take this number three grain to the milling stone by the river outside of town."

"Can I put my grain sacks in the cart and walk along with you for a while? The fastest path to the mill is through town."

"No. Master Dakor told me to have you take the two sacks along the path around the town," Subdo insisted.

Brax was disappointed because he knew they were making him take that route so he wouldn't see what they were doing at the shops. Subdo, on the other hand, seemed very happy that Brax had to carry it so far a distance.

Brax left with the two bags of grain on his shoulders. He formed the first grain bag to allow his head to be around it so both sides rested on both of his shoulders. He put the next grain sack on top so that it rested on the other bag and the top of his head. As he walked, he thought, *I definitely have to be conscious about my position with gravity.* He also decided to pay attention to his surroundings and practice the exercise he did earlier that morning. He walked slowly and found that the centered extra weight increased the fluctuations of his balance tremendously.

He finally got to the mill and knocked on the door. The mill keeper answered.

"Here is your grain to be milled," Brax said.

"Did you bring the payment to mill it?" asked the mill keeper.

"No. I was not instructed to."

"Normally, I do not ask for payment from the Cat's Claw restaurant first, but I have received no payment for milling the grain that I recently sent back to the Cat's Claw to be sold to the shops and such."

"Oh, I wondered where that milled grain came from," said Brax. "I know the Cat's Claw gets the rough grain from out of town. Sorry, I'm new to this."

"It's okay. Leave the grain to be milled. Just tell them to send a payment and I will send the milled grain as usual."

"Okay, sir. Thank you."

Brax left the grain sacks and returned to the restaurant. Lotus was waiting out front.

"Hello, Lotus. I hope you haven't been waiting long."

"No, I just did a large amount of prep work for the coming week. It will free up my time a little."

"Great," said Brax as they walked toward Lotus's house.

"How did it go? Did you learn anything?" asked Lotus.

"Not a lot, but I did learn how the grain business works for the Cat's Claw. He sent me to deliver grain to be milled. The other guys delivered the milled grain bags to the shops."

"I'm sure you'll learn more as he gets used to you," Lotus said.

It was evening when they arrived at Lotus's house, and as they started to part ways, Lotus remembered something important she wanted to tell Brax. Just as Brax turned to walk away, she grabbed his sleeve. He turned around quickly and accidentally pulled her right into his chest. He looked down and she looked up, both surprised. Brax felt his heart skip a beat. Their breath stopped and both exhaled at the same time. They both smiled widely, then started laughing.

"I'm sorry, Brax. I just wanted to tell you something."

"You can do this anytime," Brax said with a warm smile and a laugh. "What do you wish to tell me?"

"I know I mentioned tomorrow that we were going fishing for the restaurant, like when we met, but my grandmother will only watch over the restaurant tomorrow afternoon. You are not needed in the morning because Dred will be there. Master Dakor is changing the schedule a little. But this should give us more time. So, can I meet you at the pond between one-thirty and two? I'll bring a late lunch."

"That works for me. I'll be able to train longer with Master Talon in the morning."

"Great! I'll see you tomorrow afternoon. Goodnight, Brax."

"It is a good night now! Goodnight, Lotus."

As Brax walked home, he had much to think on and look forward to.

Jade Chi Do

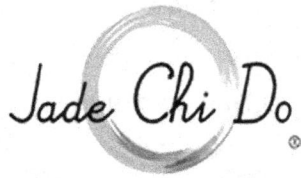

PART II - CHAPTER 11

Connections

T he next morning, Brax heard a loud chirping sound. He looked and saw a bird sitting on the windowsill. As soon as he looked at the bird, it flew away. He thought, *I have a few more minutes to sleep. The sunlight has not yet hit my face.* He had grown accustomed to using the early morning sunshine like a clock as it shone through the window onto his face.

Just before he drifted back into deep sleep, he intentionally kept himself in the gray area between sleep and wakefulness. He thought this would be the best time to practice a special exercise Master Talon taught him. In this state, he reviewed his training goals and saw them being achieved.

He then laid on his back and breathed in through his nose, filling his belly. At the same time, he opened his palms and slowly closed his right hand when he exhaled. He moved only his right hand, as he had been taught in the exercise.

In this semi-sleep state, he remembered not to move his face too much, and to only breathe through his nose. He started visualizing that he was breathing in and out through his right hand and began to feel something very powerful. The feeling of warm pressure filled both of his palms. Then he imagined breathing in and out of both palms, and something more started to happen - his breath started to disappear from his attention and he truly felt the warm pressure, or whatever it was, moving in and out of his hand as he continued to open and close it. He tried hard not to get excited and give conscious thought to it because he knew from the prior day that when he got excited, the extra experiences would just disappear.

As he continued the exercise, staying in the moment, time seemed to stop. He started using both hands and feet in the exercise, pulling his feet and toes back toward his knee caps on the inhale and back on the exhale, again following his breath. After doing all the movements several times, he stopped moving his hands and feet. He still visualized the act of breathing; the same exercise, in and out.

The moment he stopped moving and continued the exercise, he lost the feeling of the breath, and what remained was the feeling of warm pressure going inward and outward. (The warm life force.) As the feeling started to go away, he moved his attention back into his right hand, moving that hand only. He kept his other hand and his feet motionless but connected to the same visualization. By doing this, his attention on the breath began to fade away, leaving only the ebb and flow of the warm pressure feeling. This time, it was almost a magnetic feeling, like when he played with two magnets as a child. Every part of him seemed to feel this, even his forehead between his eyebrows.

Next, he was taught to do one more step, having successfully reached all the previous steps. Once all this was completed, he felt the ebb and flow throughout his body again, his spine being the center point. Just then, an overwhelming feeling of oneness overtook everything, like two vibrating tuning forks moved close to each other until one sound vibration was created. He seemed to have lost his sense of time. Then something very wondrous started to happen. The sunlight hit his face, distracting him from the moment. At the same time, the light seemed to go deeper within himself, and he completely woke up.

"Wow! That was amazing!" he said to himself. He had practiced this before but had not achieved the same effects. He realized that what had just happened was the product of all his training with Master Talon - a cumulative effect - and that it would continue to evolve, revealing itself more and more the longer and more dedicatedly he maintained his practice. Master Talon had said it would affect other parts of his training and life activities, and it was. He was more curious than ever about where this training would lead, and how it would show itself in his other arts and interests.

Brax got ready and walked to his morning training with Master Talon. He arrived at the shop to find him by the tree out front, moving in a very slow, graceful way, without any breaks in the motion. At first, he thought it was another style he had seen before, but the movement wasn't the same; it seemed more flowing, but in odd directions. He thought it must be another Jade Chi Do exercise. He also noticed that there were a few birds flying around him and a couple walking in front of him. As he got closer, still watching Master Talon, it seemed that the sun reflected off of him for a split second, like a bright burst of light on a shiny surface. Just as he gave attention to this, it instantly disappeared, and he thought, *This is like the lesson Master Talon taught me where I could not see my nose.* *

As Brax approached, Master Talon stopped and turned toward him.

"Good morning, Master Talon."

"Good morning, Brax."

"It sure is a sunny day!" said Brax.

"Yes, It is, and it is very bright to the eyes." Brax remembered the bright sun on his face that woke him earlier that morning.

"Master Talon, when I walked up to you as you were practicing, I noticed some birds around you. I couldn't help but notice they seemed to have no fear even though they were very close to you. They were just going about their business as usual. Can you explain this, please?"

"Brax, when our innermost intentions align with our outer-most being, nature is influenced in some way. Connecting your whole being to that which is around and within you with unwavering confidence creates a chain of events that seek to achieve your aligned desire. In other words, our intentions are translated into events to help achieve that which we have put out as a need. In this training, our reality is expanded. That is all I can say at the moment. This is a lesson for another time. In short, if you align with nature, then nature will seek to align with you."

Master Talon gave Brax a moment to reflect on that, then asked, "How did everything go yesterday?"

"I'm working for Master Dakor after my shifts at the restaurant. I feel it will be safer to find out more about his plans. Lotus suggested it."

"Smart girl," Master Talon said.

"Master Talon, does it have to do with the movements you were doing when I walked up? Can you show me how to do that?"

Forms were something Brax could relate to from his past martial art styles. He knew forms were important because they included groups or sets of movements done repetitively so that the body could access them without thought in time of need.

Master Talon seemed a little distracted by Brax's question. "Not today, Brax. The movements come later. We must keep working on the inner part. Without first feeling and truly defining that which has been hidden within you, in part or in full, the moves are just moves, whether it be martial arts, dancing, or anything else. Now, let's start your Jade Chi Do training."

Master Talon continued, "I will share something with you that my teacher shared with me. This truth has been the glue that has given me the opportunity to propel the growth of many students into heights only imagined by most. He taught me that these unique teachings and connected moves are attached with a sort of wave or vibration, like a musical note carried from the teacher to the student. And similar to a shared musical note, it can be replicated and become tangible. By this, the song is heard and felt in this world, our current paradigm. I know I am speaking very deeply on this subject, but as you know, I must quicken your training."

Brax could hear a pained tone in Master Talon's voice at having to accelerate his lessons so much. He knew he would have preferred to train him over time as he does with his other students, with much less talking and more special exercises to naturally take the blinders off. This ensures proper digestion and attention to each student's particular needs. Brax felt very humbled and honored that Master Talon made all this extra effort on his behalf.

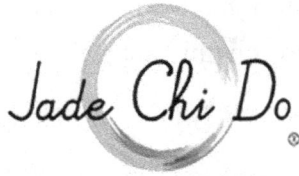

PART II - CHAPTER 12

4bolt - The Spark

"**C**an I ask another question?" Brax said.

With a smile, Master Talon replied, "You just did." Brax laughed. "But yes," Master Talon continued, "I have allowed you to ask more questions than most because it helps me accelerate you."

"I appreciate it, Master. Yesterday, I saw a board with four bolts and five springs. Tessa said Master Blade called it a 4bolt* and used it often. Do you know what this is?"

"I am happy to tell you. For today, coincidentally, we will be using such a board in our lesson. As you know, Jade Chi Do teaches a unique meditation. There is a special side of it, beyond just achieving great health. You will need to practice methods that accelerate the transfer of force physically and through the warm force. The Jade Chi Do 4bolt board can help you advance more quickly."

"Is this not combat?" Brax asked. "You said you weren't going to teach me combat."

"Because you already have this background, we must bring you to the next level in the mixture of martial arts you have. You're right - I am not here to teach you combat, but this 4bolt exercise helps create harmony of the powerful force within us. Jade Chi Do will amplify any style, and the 4bolt is one of the tools we use. Again, it is not just the movement. Reflect upon what I mentioned to you earlier about movements when you asked me to teach you the exercise I was doing this morning."

"I understand that it is beyond the movements," said Brax. "In many martial styles, movements are taught from the outside in, but we learn the movements from the inside out."

"Correct," said Master Talon. "This new exercise will reflect and show itself in all your previous styles and actions, not just this action that I am about to teach you. In combat, the student draws from a variety of combative training techniques in his repertoire. He learns these by executing repetition, which is the mother of reflex. In combat, or in life's challenges, the goal is on-demand reaction without having to stop and think. That said, including imagination and visualization in training increases this ability because they are the most effective ways to communicate one's needs to the innermost serving self. The practice of Jade Chi Do increases this tremendously. The Jade Chi Do 4bolt Board is an external tool for achieving this. In short, doing this exercise on the physical side will teach the body efficiency and economy of motion. It teaches the student to become efficient and instinctive in his reactions, and to use the correct technique from the hundreds of movements in his mental and physical memory banks. With normal training, it would take very long to go through each movement, but you can teach the body this with the use of the 4bolt board, and your body will translate this efficiently to all. The more you train and get better at it, the more your body will interpret and apply what it learns to your diverse collection of combative movements. Jade Chi Do works on reflex action, as well as the awareness to see an impending combative action against you. If you just have the awareness without the learning aspect of 4bolt, you may not have an effective response to the incoming move. In short, the sooner you perceive the action at its inception, the more time you'll have to effectively react with your trained response. Jade Chi Do training also provides to the self the most efficient way to transfer the warm force."

Brax sat quietly for a minute, meditating on all this new information.

"Come this way," said Master Talon.

They walked through the shop into the rear garden, past the training area, and to the far corner of the compound. On a tree, mounted at about shoulder height, was a Jade Chi Do 4bolt board. Brax went over and pushed on it. It was not very hard to collapse.

Brax was thinking about their earlier conversation, and his interest in learning forms*, and said. "I apologize if I seemed to want to learn physical forms first. It is just how I have been trained in all my arts."

"No problem, Brax. This is normal. Many of my students come to me looking forward to learning forms to accelerate their own style, but forms are just movements learned through muscle memory; a mixture of techniques that give the student choices to draw from when they're needed. Many teach forms in a certain order. As I said before, all arts are mixed styles to some degree. This adds more weapons to choose from. Jade Chi Do helps create a clear path to the techniques you already know and train. This is why it can be applied to anything, not just martial arts. The ability to perform any other action can be improved by it. That said, I do teach movements to increase one's continuity, or connection with oneself, by stripping away our unknown restrictions - our blinders. We then access more by our sheer dedication to the training. Due to this, one's abilities in games, business, general meditation, or combat will only increase with dedicated training."

"How did Master Dakor hit so hard with just a slap?" asked Brax. "It was soft at first, as if his palm was just touching me, but it resonated within me like a bell ringing and I dropped."

"You will learn, Brax. Let's break down your first 4bolt exercise. If a link in a chain is missing or weak, it won't work as efficiently. We must make sure your chain - the system I am teaching you - is complete and strong. Now, about Master Dakor - his slap seemed light but carried much power that seemed to penetrate further through your body, so much so that you were surprised and knocked to the ground, correct?"

"Yes, this is true."

"The 4bolt tool has two immediate goals, the first being the correct chain reaction of the body to produce maximum physical energy; and second, to provide a focused pathway for your warm force to follow using your intention. Once you have practiced this a great deal, your body will translate both parts to show itself in all the diverse, reflexive movements you have learned from your prior styles."

"I usually introduce this to students after they secure a certain definition and confidence with the warm force. In your case, due to your impending conflict with Master Dakor, I am teaching you this before this process is completed. You are still processing and defining the warm force. When completed, it will be as if the apple becomes the apple and the orange remains an orange. At first, every student's blinders attach it to a description and sense that they are already familiar with. You call it a warm pressure. Once your blinders come off, it will not feel like that, but it will feel like what it is - the warm force."

"What goal do I have?" asked Brax.

Master Talon looked at Brax and thought for a second. He wanted to get to the lesson, but he knew much more explanation was needed before he could help him progress.

"This coming goal will be difficult or nearly impossible if you have not continued to practice the warm life force training I have shared with you so far. At this point in your training, this has defined itself in part as what you described as a feeling of warm pressure, but soon it will become its own definition. Once this happens, the training I give you to direct it will truly work better for you.

I normally wait until this first goal is complete before we go to the goal I'm talking about now, but we don't have time for that. We must keep your full attention on the first goal. Afterward, with further training, you will be able to give your inner intention instructions to use this new sense. As you already know, this sense has always been within you."

"I think I understand," said Brax. "To best complete the full 4bolt exercise you are teaching me, I must continue our prior exercises. This will help me continue to refine this sense, lift my blinders to this warm force, and commune with it. I am now learning to direct it. Is this my goal now with 4bolt? How do I begin?"

Master Talon continued, "Your goal at this moment is to be open to this feeling. Go further than just visualization. Include your imagination. It is a tool that communicates with the part of you that is there to help. At this moment, your goal is to feel yourself draw in the warm force deeply as you breathe in through your feet, just like you have been doing from the beginning in the other exercises and lessons. Feel this warm force traveling in from your feet and out from your palms at the moment of the climactic end of the physical chain reaction."

Master Talon could see Brax was trying to digest everything he had just heard, and knew he had to tie it all together for him somehow, so he asked a question to help him connect this to his accelerated training. "Brax, in the Heaven and Earth exercise, when you start to straighten your legs, what is happening at that moment?"

"I am breathing out that warm pressure feeling, seeing it from within, flowing into the earth and out of my hands, in whatever direction the exercise requires," Brax replied.

"Very good! This is the flow that you're achieving in this first 4bolt exercise," said Master Talon.

"What should I feel when this first 4bolt exercise is done correctly?"

"When you feel this pulse, you will feel a kind of spark at the end. The exercise has two important parts - the physical part, and the use of the warm force. Its use creates what we call the spark. It is when the chain and the warm force work in unison at precisely the same time, yet the warm force continues to move further to the degree of your intentions, meaning going past your hand into what it is hitting or even touching. This is how Master Dakor was able to knock you down even though he seemed to just place his palm on you. He turned his entire intention toward sending it into you. He could have caused more harm but his intention was to use the cold force to feed on your broken confidence and replace it with current and future fear. I'm not saying one should not use this tactic in battle. Again, we must not look at it as a good or evil force. That said, the warm force works for a quick end. It can be merciful and preemptive when necessary. It can defuse a bad situation. It can be linear and decisive. The cold force, on the other hand, thrives and feeds on prolonged pain and fear. It keeps you treading water by breaking your confidence. This by itself slows the flow of the warm force. The cold force feeds on outside forces while the warm force feeds first from within, then outwardly."

Brax meditated on this for a long moment, then asked, "How can I know I will succeed with my training?"

"I will share a key that will help you succeed and accelerate. It will separate you from the many who never achieve. The key is this: One must continue to practice even through periods of time when you feel you're going nowhere. From this act alone, you are communicating your desire to remove your blinders. This ensures success in discovering that which has been there waiting for you all along. We must start our 4bolt training exercise now, Brax."

Allowing Brax to ask so many questions delayed the day's lessons.

"I have chosen a 4bolt exercise. We will call the first one "the spark". There are many 4bolt training exercises I can teach you after you get proficient with the first one. The number-one goal with the 4bolt is to feel and maintain a complete spark throughout the exercise. This is a feeling of open attention to the flow of the warm force, extending beyond the end of the completion of the physical chain action."

"Stand in front of the 4bolt, a little less than a complete arm's distance away, with your feet shoulder-width apart. Next, put one of your legs a foot forward. Keep both knees slightly bent. Be sure to feel balanced. Place your palm on the board with your elbow slightly bent. Next, as you are in the zone, on the inhale, bend your elbow and your legs just enough so that your hand does not leave the 4bolt board. Next, on the exhale, push but straighten your legs and arms slightly, without locking them out. Allow the push to travel physically, starting with your back foot, with each muscle activating in order, like a chain from the foot to the palm on the 4bolt board, and like whipping a wet towel."

"This is a powerful exercise for training your body. But the next step is a key that creates that which separates you from the rest, as many never get further than this point. This by itself is rewarding, but there's much more. Use your warm force to transfer through this chain. When you achieve a complete spark, the feeling will seem to be in slow motion, even though the action only takes a split second. At this speed, even though it will seem to be in slow motion, the only way to steer it is to see this motion in action or reaction to the desired completion. As you practice, you will steer your current actions and have more control of the extent and depth of the use of this warm force, which will follow your intentions. With continued work, in all of your training, you will also be able to control where your projection of the warm force ends, including past the hand. The purpose is not just to break the third brick down, it is what you felt when Master Dakor slapped you, as you described it. Just as the location of the sword is controlled by the person wielding or swinging it, one's confident inner intentions wield the warm force."

Master Talon could see that Brax was a little confused but eager to start practicing. Brax nodded, indicating he was ready to train.

"Brax, I know this is complex and difficult to understand completely right now. Not teaching this to you over a much longer period of time has been a challenge for me, but as you know, we don't have much time. This will become even more clear as you review your lessons and apply your practice of Jade Chi Do."

Seeing Brax was a little overwhelmed, he decided to change the subject by asking, "Do you have any questions about anything else?"

"Master Talon, there's something I've always been curious about. The masters, businessmen, and elite athletes who come to your shop bring a vase and take another from the shelf as they leave. Why do they do this?"

"They connect the training to the vase when they come back. They take another if they demonstrate the use of the lesson. If they haven't, they keep the vase until they do. It is a little more complicated, but I will share more as we go forward."

"Brax, go practice The Spark 4bolt exercise, then I will teach you the second exercise with the 4bolt called **Pinwheel** before you leave."

Brax did so. He felt a little discouraged when he was done so he went to Master Talon and said, "I am having a hard time gathering a good spark with the board."

"Your next lesson will help this," Master Talon assured. "It is called **Pinwheel.** Stand in the 4bolt position and allow your fingertips to touch the board, with the palm not touching the board, maintaining minimal tension in your body. Think of a circle, and within that circle is a spinning pinwheel. Visualize and imagine that you are attaching your energy to its outermost edges as it continues to spin. This builds a rhythm. Visualize this when practicing and allow it to grow in power. Next, the secret is to jump on to the spinning arms of the pinwheel. What would happen if you were to jump on a big wheel spinning around?"

"It would spin me off and throw me into the air," Brax replied.

"That's right. This brings us to the next step. When you are ready, change your attention, attaching it to the spinning energy, starting at your rear foot. Allow no breakage of the spinning of the pinwheel. Allow the energy to travel to your hand, but still visualize the pinwheel continuing to spin after you hit the 4bolt board with your palm. To practice, allow it to recharge and repeat the impact in the same way. When imagining and visualizing, this is very powerful and teaches the body not to be distracted by the distribution of energy. This will translate to all bodily movements. This is the pinwheel exercise.

Excited, Brax said, "I understand much better now. Thank you! I wish I could keep practicing but I must go now to meet Lotus."

"Okay, Brax, we must work on connecting to your awareness and reacting in this slow-motion zone. When you practice the walking exercise as you go, add one more activity: pay attention to each step - the moment your foot leaves and returns to the ground as you walk. Take note of what you feel and discover."

Brax nodded and left to go see Lotus. On his way to the Cat's Claw, he first started practicing his attention as he walked, choosing to see a spot ahead of him in the middle of the path. Next, he watched everything, using his whole peripheral vision. Then he included his breath work and added moving his breath in and out his palms. He thought, *I must just open my vision enough to see, simply bearing witness to the very moment that my feet touch and leave the ground.* At first, it was more of a distraction to Brax and pulled him away from his walking. He wished he could see it in slow motion as he had for a short time the day before.

He continued to practice, remembering his master's words - that those who keep going and never give up are the ones who get results. All of a sudden, for a fraction of a second, everything was in slow motion. In his perception, his steps felt as if they were almost floating, giving a great sense of ease of movement. It only lasted seconds, but it was enough to open the possibility. He felt a sense of excitement as he realized, *Once a true possibility reveals itself, then the confidence of it happening becomes reality.*

He wondered if this exercise would lead to what he remembered when he watched Master Blade walk away with a vase in his hand, on the path leaving Master Talon's shop.

As he looked ahead, he saw Lotus standing by the pond.

* 4bolt: To get plans to build your own Jade Ch Do 4bolt, go to http://www.4bolt.com

* Form: a set of connected movements.

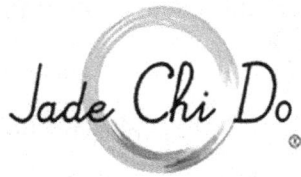

PART II - CHAPTER 13

Discovery

Lotus noticed Brax, then started to walk across the path into the field, toward the tree where Master Talon had trained with him the other day. She was carrying a big basket. *That must be the food for our picnic,* he thought. Now that his mind was on Lotus, he couldn't practice his walking exercise any longer. Lotus turned and looked at him walking toward her.

"You're right on time, Brax."

"I'm happy that I am. It gives me more time with you," he replied.

"I'm happy you are too. It's such a nice day."

They both sat by the tree, using its shadow to stay in the shade.

"How was your training today?" she asked.

Brax was quiet for a second, then replied, "Master Dakor is aware of the warm life force and has access to it, yet he chooses to feed it with the use of the cold force. Master Talon has to talk a lot in order to train me quickly, so I have to pay very close attention. It has been a challenge because he doesn't usually bombard his students with information so quickly. Besides, I usually do much better with just physical training. But I understand why he talks so much. He has taught me a great deal. Without gaining a perspective beyond my own - that is, how I see things - how else could I have grown beyond what I was before I learned anything from him? I didn't know how much I didn't know. I suspect that's true of just about everyone."

"I know you'll do well. My father told me learning happens faster when we push past our own impatience and keep practicing, because we never know how close we really are to what we're training for. In fact, most people fail when they're about to succeed, so if we stop, we only hurt ourselves. We never reach our goals if we quit. The champions of the world are the ones who push themselves past where everyone else stops."

"Your father's wisdom never stops impressing me," Brax said.

"Thanks. Let's eat!" Lotus replied.

As they sat and enjoyed the lunch she packed for them, Brax couldn't stop noticing a mark on the lower left side of her neck near her shoulder, which was revealed by the way she was sitting.

"May I ask what that mark is?" he asked. "It looks like a picture."

Lotus's smile fell and she looked sad for a second, then she said, "I will share something with you that very few people know, and you must not tell anyone. My father made me promise."

"I promise," Brax said.

"My father adopted me. My actual father and mother died when I was four. I don't remember it because I was too young. My father said my birth parents gave me this mark. He said I was very precious to them. He also said this symbol had a couple of meanings. One of them is *precious jewel,* as my parents called me. I don't know anything else about it. I have been with my father ever since."

"Maybe you will find out one day," said Brax.

"Maybe so. Now that I'm older, I may learn more from my father."

Brax looked up at the branches of the magnificent old sugar maple tree they were sitting beneath and said, "You made a good choice to sit here. The shade is perfect. It's a great place for a picnic."

"Yes, it's a beautiful tree. I was told my mother loved it. This is where my birth parents met."

"Well, then this is not only a nice spot, it's a sacred one," said Brax.

"Yes, and we didn't meet far from here either," said Lotus with a warm smile.

Brax looked into her eyes. She looked deeply back into his, and this time she didn't look away. He felt like time stood still again. After a few moments, Lotus smiled and joked, "Maybe we should say something."

Brax replied, "Oh, I think we're speaking volumes, don't you?"

"Yes, I've never felt so comfortable with anyone. It's like we can speak without even saying a word." They laughed, then Lotus added, "Can I show you something."

"Sure."

Lotus stood up and walked to the back side of the tree. Brax followed her. She pointed to a big, round rock about a meter in height. It was resting against the base of the tree. It had the same mark on it that Lotus had on her neck.

"My father told me this is the spot where my parents' ashes were spread. They were going to build a home here by this tree."

"The mark on the stone is the same as yours," said Brax.

"I noticed that. I'm not sure why."

"Perhaps it is more than just a mark given as a gift to you," he suggested.

"Maybe. My father hasn't told me anything about it, and when I ask, he says he will tell me more later, but later never arrives."

Brax reassured her, "Master Blade must have his reasons."

They continued to talk until it was almost dark and Brax said, "It's getting late. I should walk you home."

He knew she didn't like walking home in the dark, especially by herself. As they walked back to her house, Lotus's hand brushed up against his. Without thinking, he turned his hand and held hers.

"The moon is bright tonight," Lotus said, looking up into the heavens.

"Yes, it is," Brax agreed, but he was more interested in the moon's light on her flawless, radiant skin. She sensed his gaze and looked at him. As if they shared one thought, they stopped walking and turned to face each other. He took her other hand, pulled her close, and kissed her. He had longed for that moment for a long time and knew it would be exhilarating, but it was much, much more, for at that moment, he felt something more than he had ever felt before, a rush of oneness that seemed to blend both of their souls, like two notes played in tune, making their vibrations one harmonious tone. Lost in the moment as he was, Brax didn't know that this intensity was magnified by his growing mastery of the warm life force. It is love that gives life, for without it, the unit of energy of life would not exist. At that moment, everything slowed down. All was illuminated. Her heartbeat against his. Her warm breath against his neck. The velvety softness of her skin. The soft, delicate scent of her perfume. They hugged as if they were being pulled together magnetically, by a force even stronger than themselves.

As they started to walk again, Lotus said, "Brax, what was that I felt from you? I've never experienced a hug like that before. It was like we blended together. There was no you and me anymore; no separateness, for that moment. Did you feel it too?"

Brax was relieved to hear this because he felt exactly the same thing but was afraid to say it, fearing she would think he was crazy if he tried to explain it to her.

"I don't know," he replied, "but as I kissed you, the moment I touched your lips, I felt my entire self connecting with you, like we fell into each other deeply, like mixing two colors to make one."

"Have you ever felt this way before?" asked Lotus.

"Never."

Lotus smiled and walked ahead as they continued toward her house. Brax couldn't take his eyes off her.

"I can feel you looking at me," said Lotus, laughing a little. She turned to look at him. Brax felt warm and just smiled.

"Tonight, you are my moonlight. Your glow is as sparkling as when we skipped those rocks on the pond during the big full moon. My eyes cannot stop looking at such radiance," said Brax.

They arrived at Lotus's house. "This is your stop," said Brax.

"I have never invited you in, but I'd like to now. Would you like to come in?"

Brax smiled and walked in. Lotus lit a few candles. "Can I get you a cup of water?" she asked.

"That would be great."

Lotus brought two glasses of water over and sat down next to him on a long bench. Then she said, "Master Dakor is going to have you deliver some grain for him. It seems he likes seeing you carry the grain as the other two use the wheel cart to deliver the grain bags. He said Subdo would be doing your work here."

"That's strange. Why use me in the day when he could use Subdo?" wondered Brax.

"I don't know," Lotus continued. "Maybe he is using you to do jobs in locations, where he is not extorting shopkeepers until he feels he can trust you,"

Brax noticed the candlelight flickering in her eyes. It gave him a hypnotic feeling. Lotus looked back. "It seems we are talking without words again," she said with a soft smile.

"If so, I hope the conversation lasts forever," said Brax, smiling back.

Very softly, Lotus replied, "Then let's talk some more."

They both became quiet and just looked into each other's eyes for some time. After a few minutes of silence, Lotus laughed and said, "You are a great conversationalist."

Brax laughed. "Thanks! So are you. I thought the candles would burn out before we ran out of things to say."

They kissed again and Brax wished that this moment was all there was and would ever be. He suddenly realized why so many poems and plays and operas are written about love and romance. He knew, more deeply than he had ever known anything, that love is life's purpose.

"Well, I should go now," he said, though he was hoping Lotus would ask him to stay.

"You're right, Brax. You have some tough work tomorrow carrying the grain bags."

"Okay," Brax said, standing and walking to the door. Lotus impulsively ran over, almost jumped into his arms, and kissed him again.

"I will see you tomorrow, Brax."

"Then I am the richest man on earth," Brax replied. "Goodnight, Lotus."

Brax walked home full of excitement from the beautiful day he had with Lotus. He also reflected on his day's training with Master Talon and thought, *I must train with all my heart because I don't want anything to happen to Lotus.* But this thought didn't make him feel afraid, it made him angry; angry that anyone had the power to taint his joy on what was probably the best day he had ever had. He pushed away the anger, remembering that this is what Master Dakor would use to control him. Extreme anger would muddle his thoughts, and now more than ever, he needed to be crystal clear..

Jade Chi Do

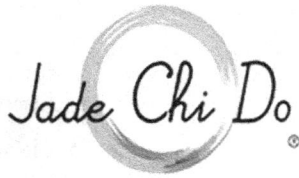

PART II - CHAPTER 14

To Achieve Outcome

Brax woke at sunrise the next morning and arrived early at Master Talon's Shop to see another master leaving with a vase in hand. He thought, *Master Talon is starting early this morning too.*

He was hoping he could talk him into starting his training earlier than usual. He walked into the shop and noticed that the vases on the shelves were dusty. Keeping them clean was one of his jobs so this bothered him. Even though he wanted to start training, he started dusting and polishing them. As he was finishing, Master Talon walked in.

"Good morning, Brax."

"Good morning, Master Talon," Brax said, setting the dust cloth down.

"It is good that you came in extra early," said Master Talon.

"I'd like to take credit for coming in early to clean these vases, but I actually came in to train more," Brax said with urgency in his voice.

"Ah, but what did you choose to do first?"

"I chose to dust."

"So indeed the credit does go to you, and I give you thanks. Even though your original intentions were different, ultimately it is the decided action that truly overrules one's regrettable prior decisions. If we live in the past, we may trip in the present. Where does this put our future? So your present decision was good! This will affect your future."

Brax reflected on Master Talon's words as they walked to the backyard training area.

"Brax, I am going to add to the Heaven and Earth exercise. These extra steps will increase the sensitivity and help finish defining the warm force as its own definition. You need to fully recognize this new sense as what it is, the warm life force. Once this happens, the lessons on how to direct and interact with it will become more achievable. Do you remember the full Heaven and Earth exercises I taught you a few months ago?" *

"Yes, Master Talon. I practice it every day," said Brax. "I've also been practicing the 4bolt exercise during my work breaks using Master Blades 4bolt board on the back-alley wall."

"Good. Let's begin. Show me the complete Heaven and Earth exercise," said Master Talon.

Brax began by first grounding himself, standing with his feet shoulder-width apart. On the start of his inhale, he lifted just his arms, like wings. At that same moment, he visualized his attention on inhaling what he called warm pressure, moving up from the earth through his legs, his palms drawing from around himself. Next, he started to exhale as he began to slowly lower his arms to his sides. At that same moment, he visualized with intention the warm pressure flowing out of his hands and down his legs into the earth.

Next, he started the Heaven and Earth exercise, including the knees bending on the inhale, with all motions flowing and in slow motion. This triggered him to get into the zone of mind that Master Talon taught him throughout his training. He then went on to practice all three sections of the Heaven and Earth exercise.

After Master Talon watched him do this a few times, he said, "Brax, I'm going to show you a training partner exercise, and how this intensifies and increases your sense of the warm force, especially when done with your teacher. We will be doing the Heaven and Earth exercise facing each other. I want you to see yourself as just being the mirror to my movements. Include the mind mirror exercise you used in my prior lessons and the special way I taught you to visualize, including your breath, until the warm force becomes the main intention. This is a different application but you will see and feel much."

The moment Master Talon started to practice while facing him as if he was the mirror, he felt like he was in a zone like no other. Again, time ceased to exist. He could feel the flow of the warm pressure. They did the full normal exercise several times until Master Talon ended it.

"That was good, Brax. Due to your dedicated practice so far, and by this exercise I just did with you, I know your sensitivity is ready to go to the next level."

Brax was proud to hear this because he knew if the student didn't practice the beginning lessons with an empty cup and full dedication and commitment, the next level would be unattainable; and if that were the case, jumping ahead to learn something would be useless.

"Now it is time to start massively increasing your awareness of this warm force," said Master Talon. His master's voice was always reassuring to Brax, but he heard something more in it at this moment. It was full of confidence in him, and it gave him a feeling of certainty about what was ahead.

"This added exercise works on creating a stronger sensitivity to the warm force. Be sure to follow the movements exactly, especially the position of the hands. I am going to add a movement to each of the three main sections of Heaven and Earth. You must keep up your regular practice of this exercise. Today's added lesson is the gateway into directing this warm force. The next section I will be teaching you is called **Heaven Moves Earth.** This exercise is an important bridge to the next. Without today's lessons, you cannot start this or benefit greatly from the next section. This is why it is so important to have a good foundation, starting with your prior training, including the Heaven and Earth exercise. It was your road to the bridge I'm teaching you today. Without a road to the bridge, the bridge cannot help you continue forward. Do you understand, Brax?"

"Yes, it is even more clear to me now. I must not expect results without practicing and assimilating what you call the road."

"Very good, Brax. This exercise is called **The Bridge.** Now, let's get to your training. Do you remember last week's lesson, when I taught you the added move to the first part of Heaven and Earth?" *

"Yes, I have included this in my training as well," Brax replied.

Hearing this, Master Talon nodded approvingly. He assumed he had because he felt a stronger sensitivity from Brax as he tested him.

"Start the first part of the Heaven and Earth exercise with the added movements, just as I taught you previously. The second part is the middle section of Heaven and Earth."

As Brax finished the first part, with his hands finishing down by his legs, he started raising his arms for part two. He then started the normal movements of the middle section of the exercise.

Master Talon continued, "The third time, as your elbows drop to your sides, and with your palms still facing outward, instead of your palms moving outward, move them forward in front of you just enough so that both hands are partly turned toward each other."

"Turn your palms slightly forward-facing so that they are not facing each other completely. Keep your hands at shoulder height and do not go any further past the front of your chest."

"Continue to breathe out and visualize the warm force flowing out of your hands and feet. You will feel a stronger warm pressure in your hands, discovering the warm force."

"Next, before you go to part three of the normal Heaven and Earth exercise, at the end of the exhale in part two, begin to inhale, drawing the warm force in. At the same time, raise your hands, facing outward, moving above your head, elbows still bent a little, with the elbow looking slightly like the letter C. Keep your palms facing up, fingers pointing and moving toward each other, ending above your head. The middle fingers are almost touching. The palms are flat and facing up, flat enough so it could hold a flat pan."

"Next, continue the normal Heaven and Earth exercise. Start expanding by pushing upward. The elbows start to unbend and straighten, but the palms stay in the same position - again, facing up and together, visualizing and directing the warm force to heaven and at the same time seeing the warm force push through your legs to your feet to the earth."

"That completes the normal Heaven and Earth exercise. Now we will add the bridge to the third part. Fittingly, it is the third time you will do the exercise. As your elbows drop, your palms end up above your head, still facing upward instead of moving straight up again. In a flowing motion, as you exhale and start to push up again, turn your palms, again keeping them mostly flat. As you rise up slowly, turn your right palm clockwise and turn your left palm counter-clockwise. Your wrist will tell you when to stop turning. Be sure not to push past that point because it will lock the wrist. You also need to stop before this or you may lose your sensitivity. The end of this upward movement will look like the letter U. Your elbows are still just slightly bent, not locked. Your arms are approximately shoulder-width apart. When your hands are at the highest point, they will still be flat, but at a slight and natural angle. If water was poured on them, it would run off on the side of the palm that has the smallest finger. Do this added bridge exercise now."

Brax did the third part while Master Talon observed. When he finished, he said, "Very good, Brax. Now do the whole bridge exercise. Remember, the added movements replace the third repeat section of each part."

Brax started the exercise. He added all three bridge additions to the normal Heaven and Earth exercise that he did daily. He felt the strongest warm pressure feeling yet and thought, *I understand now. Master Talon is teaching me contrast. I feel this added move directing this warm force in some way.*

As he started to move into the zone of his training, he felt different fluctuations. Master Talon interjected, "Brax, I am going to help hasten this and crystallize everything you've learned until now. I will do the partner exercise as I just did with you in the normal Heaven and Earth."

Brax tried not to get excited over this statement, but he was. As Master Talon stood in front of him like before, he took a deep breath through his nose, filling his belly area and holding it for about five seconds, then exhaled slowly through his mouth. At the end of the completed exhale, he held it for three seconds. He did this twice.

Brax joined Master Talon the second time as he started the bridge exercise. Brax then became the mirror, connecting his breath and using visualization from intention located deep within himself. Brax was also using the prior mind exercise, seeing all around himself without losing focus on the center.

At points, Brax felt like it was Master Talon breathing, like he was a real mirror. He noticed when he got to the added bridge exercises that he felt something very strong and wondrous. He got excited for a moment and almost lost the awareness and connection with his teacher. He had already learned that excited emotion caused the extra experience to go away very quickly, and that it was hard to recapture it.

They did the bridge exercise completely three times. After this, knowing Brax was ready, Master Talon began to intensify the exercise by alternating one regular technique and one bridge technique twice, very slowly. He did this in all three sections.

Brax felt a strange sensation, like a bubble popping. The contrast was so intense, he no longer felt the warm pressure for a few moments, and his body recognized it as its own sense without mislabeling it as anything other than the warm force.

Brax blurted out, "Just as an apple is an apple, so the warm force is the warm force!"

Witnessing and feeling this great awakening, Master Talon ended the exercise.

"Brax, what did you feel?"

With a confident smile, Brax declared, "I can confidently tell you - the warm force is like a feeling of inserting my hand into a moving river of warm life energy. It was almost like a resistance, yet at the same time, I feel the water, or warm life force, also being pulled into my hands."

The master smiled, taking real joy in his progress and excitement. "Brax, be sure to keep practicing all your prior lessons as they will express themselves in different and even more wondrous ways as you grow with continued training. I will also teach you ways to teach this, as I do. Just as I told you, my teacher had one main request, which was that I help others grow and find what they have been seeking without knowing it. Your students will find you, as you found me, but before you ever share this, be sure to give them the right recipe. To do this, you must make sure you have defined this within yourself. You must have the apple in your hand to hand the apple over, not the orange."

"I understand," said Brax.

"Now that you have walked over this bridge, only by this fact can I teach you to move the apple."

"Maybe throw the apple?" said Brax with a hinting smile.

"All in time, Brax," said Master Talon. "Doing this exercise, as well as the others I have taught you, can be accelerated not only by diet and normal exercise like walking, lifting weights, etcetera, but also by doing Jade Chi Do exercises in water. Keep your head above the water for now. When you're at a higher level, you'll do some of them completely submerged."

"I can't wait!" Brax exclaimed.

Master Talon smiled and chuckled good-naturedly at his youthful enthusiasm.

* Reference the full Heaven and Earth exercise in Part I Chapter 4

* The first part of Heaven and Earth is in Chapter 7.

Train with a teacher as you practice being the mirror.

Get free access to a beginner video, with a teacher.

Go to https://dwaynetfeeley.com/course/

Jade Chi Do

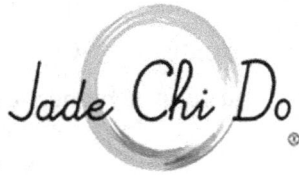

PART II - CHAPTER 15

Growth

B rax finished his morning training and arrived at work just a little late. Lotus was watching for him from the window when she saw him walking toward the restaurant.

"Did you sleep in, Brax?" she asked, smiling.

"No, I was having a deep training session with Master Talon. Good morning! How is your day going so far?"

Lotus smiled, looked into his eyes, and stole his usual line. "It's a good morning *now*."

Brax smiled and didn't say anything but gazed into the oceans of her eyes, hoping to recapture the wordless magic from the night before. Lotus knew what he was doing and played along.

"There we go again, having one of our silent conversations!" she said with a gentle laugh.

"I really think we need to talk this way more often."

"I hope so," Lotus agreed.

Over her shoulder, Brax saw Dred motion to him to come to the kitchen. He excused himself and walked over. Dred said, "Your two grain bags are ready to be delivered to the River Road grain mill, the same one you delivered to the other day. Don't go through the town. Use the same road along the river. Be back before lunchtime. I have another task to do for Master Dakor."

Brax left, again thinking it made no sense for him to take the long way while carrying heavy grain bags when he could just take the shortcut through town, especially since he needed to be back before noon. This meant he would have to move fast. *It must be that Master Dakor wants me to work harder again,* he thought. He was a little disappointed that he would be rushing too much to practice with the grain bags like he did the first time.

When he was walking along the river's edge toward the mill on the River Road, he noticed that the sky was starting to cloud up and thought a storm must be approaching. He began to meditate on Master Talon's lessons and remembered him saying he had reached the same level of sensitivity once in the past. The warm force reflected itself and slowly amplified in all areas of his life. He told Brax that no matter what one's profession or interests are, the warm force would begin to express itself in extraordinary ways. He was told not to be surprised by this, but accepting. This would help him keep his blinders down so it could continue to express itself.

He arrived at the mill a little exhausted but earlier than he expected to. When he delivered the grain, a different person answered the door and just took it with a curt thank you. As he was leaving, Brax noticed what sounded like fear in the man's voice. He thought perhaps Master Dakor or his thugs must have gotten to him. He then wondered if he had ever been paid for the prior bags from his first delivery.

Brax was walking by the river about halfway back to the restaurant. He was ahead of schedule so he decided to sit by the water and meditate for a few minutes. He was tired from rushing the bags there and hoped to rest for a bit. He sat on a stone about chair height by the water's edge. He remembered two special exercises taught by Master Talon. The first was about a windmill as the wind blew. He couldn't do the second lesson because it needed two things - sitting by the water while it was starting to rain. He had tried it only one time before. The sky was darkening so he figured this was the perfect opportunity.

He reviewed his lesson from memory and began the exercise. He looked about six paces out over the water and focused his vision on the center of that area. Next, he looked as far as he could to his sides with his full peripheral vision, without moving his eyes. Then he practiced seeing both the middle and sides of his vision. At first, he could tell he was focused on the middle, then he focused on the peripheral, side vision. It felt like it was one or the other. Then he remembered to just look at it with a gaze. He noticed that it was his conscious mind that was not able to see everything without going back and forth with his vision.

When he remembered Master Talon's training, he gave his full intention from within to look as a gaze, to see all. Just as he finally got into this specific zone, it started to rain. At first, it brought him out of the gaze and he looked at one drop, then the other. But he was able to return to his zone and gaze at all he saw by directing himself with his intention. He started to see all the droplets falling at the same time, but it was as if they were falling in slow motion, even the ripples. It was a powerful experience, and for a few minutes that timeless feeling returned. At the peak of experiencing this, he couldn't help but get extremely excited. That made everything return to regular speed again.

As he stood up, he knew he had achieved a much larger effect than the other times he had tried this exercise. He also knew this was due to what he achieved the day before during the partner exercise with Master Talon.

As he was lost in thought, he saw a flash of a picture in his mind's eye of someone swinging at him from behind. Simultaneously, and with lightning-fast precision, he turned and struck the attacker's arm. There was a sound like someone breaking a dry stick in half. The attacker screamed in agony. He had broken his arm with a block. The attacker regrouped and lunged again like a wounded animal, trying to hit Brax in the chin with the elbow of his other arm. Everything slowed down to super slow-motion, so much so that Brax could actually watch the elbow coming toward his chin. He again reacted quickly and instinctively based on his prior, repetitive martial arts training, deactivating the attacker's movement by striking his arm and shoulder joint. There was another sound - this time a dull pop - when the attacker's shoulder was dislocated. He hadn't blocked or redirected the second attack; he had suppressed and smothered it by striking harder and faster before the attacker could even complete his motion. Both strikes were delivered at the start of the attacker's movements, as if Brax was reading their minds. Even stranger, he felt no impact, or even contact. It was as if his strike just went through the attacker.

They both fell into the water, but both of the attacker's arms were rendered useless. Brax could see the attacker was drowning so he pulled his face above the water and dragged him to the shore. He struggled to his feet and ran off. There was another attacker staring at Brax, but after seeing what he had just done to the other two with such efficiency, and seeing the fearless resolve in Brax's eyes, he ran away like a frightened child.

As Brax watched them flee, he was amazed at how the warm force had expressed itself. He noticed that the movements he used were from a brutal martial art style he was training. It had flowed out of him naturally, like a file being selected from a library of choices. He was a little excited and also felt a sense of empowerment. He enjoyed it for a second before catching himself and realizing this was the cold force pulling on him. It was very active, as the fear the attackers felt fed his ego. This was, in part, what Master Talon described as the lure of the cold force. He knew there was a risk of bandits on the outskirts of town so he considered the attack to be random.

He walked back to the Cat's Claw restaurant soaking wet and arrived just before noon, as requested. The sun and wind had dried his clothes somewhat but he was still a sight. Dred looked very surprised to see him. Brax thought this was because he had hurried and was back sooner than expected, or perhaps his appearance. He had no way of knowing that Master Dakor had arranged the bandits to take him out and get him away from Lotus.

Dred left quickly and Lotus walked into the kitchen. "Brax, you're all wet! What happened?"

"It's a long story."

"Okay, tell me later. I'll go get you some dry clothes. My father leaves a couple of sets here for this very reason."

She opened a cabinet, took out pants and a shirt, and handed them to him.

"See you inside. Please hurry - we're getting busy."

Brax changed and went to work. As he and Lotus went about their usual business, the two attackers were meeting Master Dakor on the opposite side of town. Subdo stood behind him as he met with the two attackers.

"So did you do the job?" asked Master Dakor.

"No, we didn't. He was harder to handle than we expected," said the attacker, holding his broken arm.

"That's too bad," Master Dakor said. "Well, you still deserve to be compensated for trying. Follow me. I don't want anyone to see me paying you."

He led them into an alley and said, "Wait here."

The two stood next to a wall as Master Dakor turned around and took out his wallet, as if he were counting money. The two hit men smirked at each other, relieved they would be paid in spite of failing to kill Brax, when Master Dakor turned with lightning speed and slammed his palms into each of their chests. They both hit the wall, then stood for a moment, eyes wide, mouths open - the look all men have when they know death is upon them, like ice water had been injected into their hearts. Master Dakor looked them in the eye, feeding on the horror of their final thoughts and emotions like a drunkard gulping a bottle of booze. Then both dropped in unison, as dead as bags of sand.

Master Dakor looked at Subdo, who was also full of fear at what he had just witnessed, and pointed at the bodies.

"Get rid of these incompetents."

"Yes, sir."

Subdo dragged them away and hid their bodies behind some trash cans. Before he left, Master Dakor told him, "We need to get the emerald soon. I have a plan. I must leave soon to get more fighters, and they will need to get paid."

Subdo knew this meant more extortion from local shopkeepers. Knowing how formidable and fearless Master Blade would be when he returned, Dakor planned to have many fighters ready to show dominance, with the ultimate goal of gaining control of Master Blade and his restaurant. Master Dakor had another plan in place as a kind of insurance, and he would implement it soon.

Meanwhile, at the Cat's Claw, it was lunchtime and the restaurant was busy. Brax was cleaning the dishes as Lotus walked up and set more down.

"Wow, I've never seen it so busy," said Brax.

"It must be the weather," Lotus said. "It's always busier when it rains. Thank goodness it doesn't rain a lot here, but when it does, it really pours."

As Lotus turned to leave, she slipped and started to fall. As she fell, her arm hit a cup on the counter and it became airborne. Brax was facing away by the sink, but without looking, he turned and simultaneously caught her with his left arm and the flying cup with his right hand. They stood in a frozen moment, Lotus looking at him in amazement.

"Now *that's* a good catch!" said Lotus.

Brax was surprised too but played it off, as if he did that kind of thing all the time.

"Yes, *you* certainly are a good catch, Lotus," Brax said with a smile. She looked around to make sure nobody was watching, gave him a quick peck on the cheek, and went back to work. As he started to do the dishes, he thought about what had just happened, and again felt a surge of cold force trying to feed his ego. He thought, *This lure is stronger than I thought it would be.*

Finally, the workday was done and Brax walked Lotus home as usual. He didn't tell her what happened so he wouldn't worry her.

They walked quickly as he held her umbrella for her. When he left her at the door, she said, "I'll see you in the morning. Would you please take my umbrella?"

He did and they kissed.

"Thank you again for catching me when I fell earlier today," she said.

"I'm just returning the favor! You caught me the first day we met. When you threw the net, I might as well have been one of those fish," said Brax.

Lotus teared up a little and said, "Goodnight, Brax."

"Goodnight, my Lotus," said Brax.

He reflected on the day as he walked home. He was excited about seeing Master Talon again in the morning and telling him about what had happened. But for now, he needed rest.

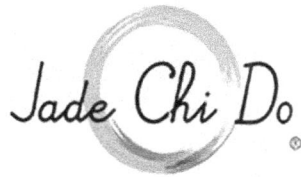

PART II - CHAPTER 16

To Heal and Hurt

B rax arrived at Master Talon's Shop the next morning and walked to the back area to find Master Talon sitting at the same table where they trained with the stones a few days earlier.

"Good morning, Master Talon!"

"Good morning! Come and sit.".

As usual, Brax had plenty of questions.

"Master Talon, as you know, being a martial artist, I'm familiar with the concept of chi. Why don't you just call this warm force that?"

Master Talon replied, "By our definition, chi is both warm and cold force, and does not teach you balance or give more meaning; thus, we go further then just the word chi. Also, we have talked about having blinders, meaning if you have a strong opinion or definition of this from another art, then just calling it chi would indeed slow or end further growth in this area of Jade Chi Do. Trained masters are especially susceptible to this because they have already formed an opinion on what chi is and so may not reach the higher level of the use of their art or profession, or discover some unknown natural gifts they have personally. In turn, by narrowly defining this with a general term like chi, you may not attain the results of what is being taught."

"I understand, Master Talon. After the training, I finally defined the warm force. This morning, I did the exercise just before waking and I could tell the difference between breath and warm force, and when I connected both. I felt myself moving warm force. It was amazing! At the beginning, I never thought it would be so intense.* I must say, the warm force truly expressed itself in many of my prior trained reflexes. I was attacked during a delivery yesterday and I reacted almost as if I knew in advance that they would strike. I reacted in a zone."

"That is good, Brax. It will only grow from here. Now, as you sit here, put your hands out and rest your elbows on the table. The next exercise I will teach you today is very important. It is called **Earthen Palm Training**. There are many variations but the original has two parts. The first is training with yourself; the second is with a partner. Now, let's work on number one."

"Put your elbows on the table, shoulder-width apart and palms up. Raise your forearms with your palm, connecting in a praying posture. Next, while your hands are still in praying fashion, raise your elbows off the table. Now lower your hands at the wrist until your elbows are pointing almost straight to your sides. Your praying hands will be right in line at about chest level. Next, move your whole praying position to the right and visualize the warm force connected with your breath, first pushing from your left palm through the right palm to the right elbow, and then pulling from the right elbow through your left palm, in reverse. The key is to direct with just your left hand pushing and pulling/inhaling. That hand and the right are just felt passively. Next, make the right hand the dominant one. With practice, you will feel and gain use of this. Practice this now."

Brax got himself into the special zone he was taught and practiced the one-person Earthen Palm exercise. He was excited as he felt this moving from his innermost intentions. Master Talon saw how well he was doing.

"Okay, Brax, let's work on something I feel is important to balance out your training.

It's called **Heaven's Hand** exercises. There are many, but the first is most important because, like all the training you have received so far, if you miss the steps of training in the beginning, you may lack what each lesson and exercise is meant to increase, and lose its total value as a result. We will start here. In battle, it is good to know how to heal, not just how to hurt."

"Still sitting at the table, turn around and sit with your body facing away. Put your left hand on your knee cap. If your knee was hurt and you needed to keep going, you would notice something very amazing. Push your hand slightly down over the knee cap. As you're pushing, breathe out of your palm and direct and extend the flow of the warm force inward into the knee, going right out of your foot."

As Brax did this, Master Talon continued, "Next, pull your hand upward, still touching your knee while you inhale the warm force up through your foot, out of your knee, and into the palm, keeping your intention on this and your knee. Connect this with your breath and keep breathing this way. You will feel the flow and the pain will lessen or disappear. This is the short term affecting the long term. Due to your focus on it, it communicates its importance. This helps optimize the natural healing process. You will be able to help others as well. My teacher could erase a bruise if he caught it right away. It was awesome to witness how quickly it disappeared. At times, it seemed immediate. Practice this when you can too," said Master Talon.

Brax did this exercise for a few minutes and could feel the flow of the warm force. Master Talon continued, "Now let's go to the back area. This is the second exercise of **Earthen Palm**, which is done with a training partner. The use of a partner speeds up the results, and even more so when done with your teacher because he can help direct you while connecting. But either way, with communication between each student, another student can learn this. It may just take longer. It is a challenge training exercise that was focused on the sending and returning of chi, designed to show the directing of the warm force part. At first, this was just a training exercise our teacher taught to me, Master Dakor, and the other student. But when we practiced it, we noticed the depth increasing. We started with the elbow as the first level of depth. We communicated that to the partner and no harm came to them. After we had gotten better with this form of partner training, we noticed something else. When one became a little angry, it could be felt in the push, just before and after it. It was like a vibration was attaching to it. The teacher warned us that this was not the goal of the exercise, and he said he would teach special exercises later on. We were also instructed to not practice the intention to attach this anger on the sending and pushing, as your training partner in this exercise helps pull as you push, learning direction and flow, as well as feeling another's push."

Master Talon went silent and serious for a moment, remembering, then continued, "It was not long before Master Dakor realized the potential of this and misused it in the local village near where my teacher taught us. He began to get addicted to the fear and control he instilled from using the cold part of the life force. As you know, he now seeks to rule over others in this way, in a much larger way, feeding his ego. This is why it's important for you to learn a deeper perception of your warm life force - the next step - when and only when you have crossed the line of the warm force having its own recognition; its own name. If this has not happened, this training will not be as rewarding as it could be. I know you have been devoted and practiced much, so I know you are ready for this. Your innermost self realizes your seriousness and is backing you up to achieve this. With diligence and confidence, much is possible."

Master Talon stood and faced Brax. "The purpose of this next exercise is to sense the push of this force, in-depth and from another. Both must be sensitive and trained in chi, as we have trained. This exercise will help define the warm force part as well as the cold part. It is a partner exercise called **The Ray of Sunshine**. To illustrate the meaning of that name, let me ask you - just as the sun comes out from behind the clouds, what does it feel like as it hits your face?"

Brax thought for a moment. "I first feel the sun as warmth on my face, then I feel the heat radiating deeply into my skin."

"Good. Would you also say that the longer you are exposed, the deeper the heat may go?"

"Yes, most definitely," Brax replied.

"This will help you see how this warm force is directed in a similar fashion, but by your innermost intention."

Brax followed Master Talon's train of thought. He realized this would help him relate to directing the warm force.

"Brax, using this inner intention this way will help you and your training partner feel the push or the pull in the gentle intensity of the warm force pushed beyond the hand."

"Okay, so it helps each student increase their control and push their warm force?" asked Brax.

"Yes," said Master Talon.

"Now, stand in front of me with your feet shoulder-width apart, arms in front of you at shoulder height, palms facing me, fingers pointing up."

Brax did so. Master Talon then placed both his hands against Brax in the same alignment, with his elbows slightly bent.

"Now breathe and direct the warm force to my palms. Just push your arms out slightly, pull back slightly on the inhale, and draw the warm force in," Master Talon directed. "I will maintain palm contact with you. I will then put my innermost intention to align with yours and follow your direction of the warm force."

Brax felt the warm force moving. It felt like a flowing river that he was directing for just a moment.

"Good, Brax. I felt the depth at the elbows. Now just relax. I will direct this for a few minutes."

Brax nodded. Within a moment, he felt movement that was both extremely powerful and smooth. It was almost hypnotizing as he followed the flow of the warm force.

When they finished, Master Talon asked, "How is your 4bolt training going?"

"Good, but I haven't practiced it since I defined and directed the warm force."

"You will notice the spark much better now, but it will still take practice to keep growing in your abilities," said Master Talon. "This brings up the next exercise. It is called **Earthen Palm**. It's a challenge exercise between two opponents. Though its roots are from practice with a training partner, as I mentioned, it has turned into a demonstration of who has the better directing ability. It engages all of one's training, from awareness to the sense you have felt at the inception of your opponent's intention to strike. The simplest definition is the ability to be one step ahead of your attacker. You can also see it as catching the gate just as it starts to blow open. If you had a large herd of cattle enclosed by a fence, and the cows were anxious to stampede once the gate was opened, wouldn't it be better if you became aware of the gate opening and closed it before it could open completely? If the gate opened wide, it would be much harder to stop the herd. You would only be able to divert it. Most do not reach the gate just as it starts to open, but many do get to the gate when it's almost half open and are able to redirect the stampede. There are many styles that teach combat from this standpoint."

"Earthen Palm has two parts - physical and internal - and they are equal to their use of the warm force. But some lean further into the cold force, using this to tip the scales, as it does take more training to go further with the warm force. Remember, the cold or warm force is not "evil" or "good" - that rests within the person's choice. Choice is like the forge and the hammer to the sword. We are the sword. The Earthen Palm Challenge is on the physical side of the 4bolt training and the use of the warm force. I will repeat myself a few times today, so you will get a clearer picture of today's important lesson. I feel Master Dakor may challenge you if he learns that I am training you in Jade Chi Do."

Master Talon thought for a moment and said, "To do this exercise, you start out in the same stance as the 4bolt Board number one exercise.* Both opponents put their hands up against each other as if it is the 4bolt board. It is dangerous to lock your elbows so keep them slightly bent. The winner stays standing. This can be dangerous, but one's own connection to the warm force of life is good when directed to protect oneself. This will also increase the spark push in 4bolt. With practice, it increases its communication."

"This is the first I have heard of this challenge," said Brax. "Could you explain just a little more so I'll be prepared?"

"Okay, but don't worry," Master Talon said. "After working with you today, I feel you will do well, as long as you don't get distracted. In the Earthen Palm Challenge, two competing individuals stand facing each other in the first original 4bolt training stance and palm exercise of 4bolt. Both put their palms up and place each on the other, as if the other is the 4bolt board. They *do not* start hammering each other first. They start by sending the warm force back and forth, like playing catch. The opposite side bends at the elbow to dissipate the force being sent, both physical and non-physical. Both students select someone to watch who will determine the winner. That person yells "start" to begin the exercise. Then each bend their arms at the elbows to absorb the force. However, if one becomes careless, the challenge is given back and the victor sends a shock of physical and non-physical force back into the body. One falls, which denotes vulnerability. Instead of fighting more and finishing off the opponent, the victor is simply the one who remains standing. It is a gentle win with no harm or cold force intentions, which can only result in more destruction. One does not hurt the other once they are on the ground. This is just a sign that the one still standing has won."

"Thank you, Master Talon. I must go to the restaurant now. I will continue all the previous exercises as usual. I know now that doing them will take on more meaning as I feel and direct the warm force."

Brax went on his way to work, with much to reflect upon about the day's lesson and exercises.

* Reference exercise chapter 11.

* Reference chapter 12 for the 4bolt Board number 1 exercise.

* To learn more on Earthen Palm, go to
http://www.EarthenPalm.com/

Jade Chi Do

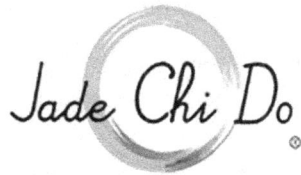

PART II - CHAPTER 17

The Surprise

When Brax arrived at the restaurant, Lotus met him before he reached the front door.

"Good Morning, Brax! My grandmother said she is watching over the restaurant for the day and Subdo is in the back, so she said we could take the day off!"

"What a nice surprise! Where are we going?"

"Just follow me," Lotus said.

"I have no problem following you, even to the moon," Brax said with a smile. Lotus looked back with a sparkle in her eyes and said, "I am sure you would."

Brax was curious to find out where they were going. He followed her for quite some time until they arrived at a river and started hiking their way up along the bank until they reached a large and spectacular waterfall. Brax thought this had to be the spot Lotus was taking him to. Just then, Lotus turned, walked to his side and said, "Isn't this a beautiful sight?"

"It certainly is!" said Brax. He then turned and looked into her eyes. "But I am looking at the most beautiful sight I've ever seen."

She blushed and said, "I meant the waterfall, silly!"

He looked at the waterfall again and said with mock boredom, "Yes, it's very beautiful too. I suppose."

They both laughed, then Lotus took Brax's hand and said, "Follow me. I have something more to show you."

As they walked closer to the base of the waterfall, Brax saw a little path in a group of trees next to the waterfall and became even more curious about where she was taking him. He followed her in and saw a cave behind the waterfall.

"My father showed me this place in case I ever needed to get away and relax. He called it his meditation spot. I wanted to show it to you because it's so beautiful and peaceful."

Brax looked at the waterfall. The sun shining through it illuminated it, making it sparkle with light, as if it were electrified.

"Let's have lunch," Lotus said. She walked him deeper into the cave to a blanket on the ground. She removed the blanket to reveal a picnic basket under it. Unbeknownst to Brax, she had prepared a meal to surprise him.

"You made this?" he asked. She smiled mischievously and nodded.

"You are full of surprises," Brax said, laughing. "Thank you for going to all this trouble."

"You're welcome! Doesn't it feel magical?"

"Yes! The lighting is amazing, and the sound of the falling water is so powerful."

She picked up the blanket and spread it on the floor, and they enjoyed a delicious meal together. Afterward, she stood and walked to the edge of the ledge, then extended her hand to touch the falling water. Brax walked over, stood behind her, and reached out to do the same. She turned to look up at him and said, "It is so beautiful, isn't it?"

"Yes, it is." He smiled, not taking his eyes off of her.

"You're just looking at me again," she said, her cheeks turning red. They kissed, then she took him by the hand. They walked over to the blanket and sat, just looking into each other's eyes.

"There we go again, talking without words," she said with a soft laugh.

Brax moved closer and said in a flirtatious way, "Let me express myself in another language."

Brax moved closer to her but she put her hand on his chest and said, "Let me show you *my* language first."

She grabbed his shirt at the shoulders and pulled it off. Brax gave her a gentle kiss as Lotus pulled him back onto the blanket. They made love in its purest sense, the roar of the waterfall echoing throughout the cave, rising and falling in rhythm with them. Afterward, they laid in each other's arms without talking, just listening to the water and absorbing the light flickering in the cave.

"Thank you for sharing this very special spot. Being with you here has been the most extraordinary and magic moment of my life," Brax said.

Lotus looked at him with warmth that only real love can convey. "I will never forget this moment, or this day."

"Neither will I," said Brax. They gently kissed again, then laid back down. When it was almost dark, Brax said, "It's getting late. We should go while there's still some light."

They left, holding hands all the way back to her house, rarely speaking or feeling the need to.

"It's fascinating how we say so much to each other yet speak so little," said Lotus.

"Yes, it is. What a wonderful day it has been," Brax agreed.

"Things seem to be going more smoothly at the restaurant too. Maybe my father will return and Master Dakor will stop his illegal activities," said Lotus with youthful naïveté.

"Perhaps. I hope so."

When they arrived at her house, Brax asked, "Do you want me to stay?"

"I would, but my father might come home and I would rather tell him about you first, if that's okay."

"Of course. That's fine," said Brax.

They kissed and he went on his way. He was very excited about the day, though his joy was again tainted with concern about what Master Dakor's ultimate plans might be.

The next morning, Brax made his way to Master Talon's shop for his training. He arrived to find Master Talon sitting in front of the shop. When he first looked at him, for a split second he again seemed to have a kind of brightness around him, even brighter than the first time he had seen this phenomenon. It appeared he was looking straight ahead, meditating in the way he had taught him to do. Brax thought, *I have so much more to learn.*

"Good morning, Master Talon."

"Good morning, Brax. Today's lesson will be short now that you're directing the warm force by visualizing from your innermost intention. Today's exercise is one that will prepare you to be ready for many lessons to come. I feel your journey has just begun. Remember, as I was taught by my teacher, I ask you now to honor the same. Teach the warm force by example. Emanate like the sun. By doing this, those who are ready will see it. In turn, help them discover that which lays waiting within them. They will find you when the time is right, when the words you write end up in their hands, or by sharing the same social sphere."

"I will, Master Talon," Brax said.

"Good. The next exercise is called **Opening the Lotus**. This is an exercise I couldn't teach you before because you did not yet have the necessary awareness of the tangibility of the warm force. If you had done this exercise earlier, you would have achieved little to no tangible value from it."

"I understand," Brax said.

Master Talon continued, "A student once asked me, 'What is tangible value?' I answered, 'If you need to ask me, you're not ready for it. It is like a recipe, and if any of the ingredients are missing, one cannot expect a desirable result. Results are earned, not given, and results without desire are hard to achieve.'"

Master Talon continued, "I am very pleased that you have demonstrated this through your practice. It reflects on the growth value of each lesson."

Brax said, "I have also discovered that when I go through the original training, it takes on a new meaning and strengthens each subsequent step, like a new lesson being done all over again. I see why it is so important to continue the original practice."

"You're right. Each time you go through the lessons, your insights, application, and sensitivity will become stronger. Applying this process, you then will know when you are ready for a new lesson."

"Is this one of the reasons the masters and others take a vase when they are given a new lesson, then return it sometime in the future when they have achieved the lesson? Is the purpose of the vase also to give them motivation to practice when they see it on their own table each day?" Brax asked.

"Yes, that is one of the reasons, in addition to the others I told you about," Master Talon replied. "Okay, that's enough questions for now; let's get to this lesson. Opening the Lotus is simple but technical, and it is achieved only if you have defined the warm force and made it tangible. Always be sure to practice this inside or in a place where there is no wind.

"Stand with your feet shoulder-width apart. Your legs should be straight but not locked. Your arms and palms are straight down on each side, with your palms flat against your sides, but not touching your sides. Next, open your arms, pulling your palms away like wings from your sides about one foot. Breathe in as I taught you in the Heaven and Earth exercise. Next, on the exhale, turn your palms outward so they are facing in front of you. Next, inhale the warm force. As you inhale slightly, pull your palms back, opening your hands a little while swinging at the elbows, like pulling a rope. Again, while doing this action, you're pulling - inhaling the warm force."

Master Talon observed carefully and was pleased to see Brax executing his instructions perfectly. He continued, "Next, push your palms forward, closing your palms with your fingers just a little. Your hands will end the forward movement, about the width of your palm, in front of your hips. Remember, the movement of your arms is mostly swinging at the elbow. Push, breathing out the warm force. If done correctly, your palms will move back and forth about the distance of half of your foot. Do this back and forth several times."

When Brax had completed this, Master Talon said, "Okay, now we'll move on to **Part Two of Opening the Lotus.** This time, while in the process of inhaling, breathe in with your nose with a full belly breath, overlapping to expand somewhat into the chest. Hold it fully and imagine that you're exhaling at the start of the motion, but not really air from your lungs; you're exhaling your warm force while still holding your full breath slightly. In your hands, you will feel the warm force leaving. Next, you will still take a full breath but imagine you're inhaling the warm force as you pull your palms back, closing your palm from your fingers slightly. If it's hard to hold a full breath, breathe very lightly and connect to the proper flow direction. By this time, you will be feeling the separation of warm force. It will feel like you're still breathing - the same feeling of the warm force flowing in through your palms and feet. The last part will help increase your ability to direct it, and learn more lessons to do so."

He paused as Brax relaxed deeply into the exercise, then said, "Next, you will need to breathe, exhaling out of your mouth. Then start the Opening the Lotus exercise again while breathing and connecting as usual. Then do the second part again. Then go back to the first part. Make sure you're breathing enough air. Your body will tell you. The main purpose is to increase the volume of the sense and use of the warm force over the volume of the sense of breath. By doing so, it increases its expression in all your activities. It also increases my ability to teach you more exercises to further discover and direct the uses of the warm force. Now practice this," said Master Talon.

Master Talon said he would be back in a little while and went into his shop. Brax practiced the Opening the Lotus exercise diligently. After some time, Master Talon returned, watched Brax practicing for a moment, and said, "Good form. You can stop now. What did you get out of this exercise so far?"

"Just after I held a full breath and continued as if I was breathing out, though without actually breathing out yet as you instructed, my hands really felt the warm force flowing out. When I went to breathe in, again without *actually* breathing in, my hands and feet felt the flow of the warm force coming in. It was strange . . . when I was in that moment, it was like I was really breathing too. Then I went back to breathing with the warm force and I could feel both processes as different yet connected, when I chose to."

"Good, Brax! Your continued practice will be rewarded by even greater ability," said Master Talon.

"Thank you, Master. I must go to work now. May I leave?"

"Of course. Have a good day. I will see you at tomorrow's training."

Brax went on his way to work, more excited than ever about his training and rapidly expanding abilities.

Jade Chi Do

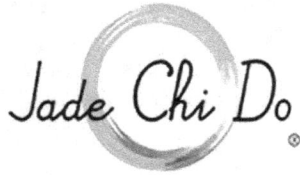

PART II - CHAPTER 18

An Uncommon Day

Brax arrived at the restaurant and, as usual, immediately looked for Lotus, but she was nowhere to be found. He saw her grandmother, Tessa, in the corner with her head down.

"Good afternoon. Do you know where Lotus is?" asked Brax.

"She went to see her aunt," she answered sadly.

Brax thought, *She must miss her a lot to be so sad.*

Before he could ask any more questions, Master Dakor yelled from the back of the restaurant, "Brax, come here!"

Brax walked over and Master Dakor said, "Deliver this grain sack. You'll be going to a local cabin just outside the city."

When he was given the directions, he remembered the night when he got on the roof and listened to Master Dakor's meeting. It was the same location he had heard him say then.

"Don't go in. Just knock and set the grain bag down on the porch near the door. I will be leaving this morning for a meeting. I'll be back in two days. I'm traveling a couple of towns away to hire a few more employees of my choice."

Brax delivered the sack as instructed. As he dropped it on the porch, part of it opened and he saw money mixed with the grain. He thought, *Hmm. I wondered where the money was going. That explains it.*

Brax left to go back to the restaurant. He got down the path a little and started practicing his teachings while paying attention to his peripheral vision when he noticed a scarf to his right at the base of a tree. It was on the opposite side of the tree so he hadn't seen it on his way to the cabin. He picked it up and thought, *This looks like Lotus's silk scarf.* He then smelled it, recognized her perfume, and said, "This *is* her scarf!"

He wondered how it had gotten there. He thought, *It's so close to that cabin, and this part of the path ends there. She must be there. I must see inside. I'll just act like I'm delivering more grain.*

Brax made it back to the cabin and knocked on the door. A voice from within shouted, "Who is it?" Brax immediately recognized the voice as one of the people who met Master Dakor in the alley when he was eavesdropping from the roof.

"It's the Cat's Claw grain delivery," Brax answered.

The voice yelled out, "One was already delivered a half hour ago."

"I have another."

The man opened the door, but as soon as he saw there was no bag, he tried to strike Brax. Brax slipped the punch and hit him hard on the jaw, knocking him unconscious. He then tied him up inside the cabin. He looked around for Lotus and heard a faint, muffled sound coming from a wooden storage box at the back of the room. He quickly opened it and saw Lotus inside, bound and gagged. He pulled her out and quickly untied her. She hugged him and said, "Brax . . . thank you. I hoped you were going to save me."

"Are you hurt?" he asked.

"No, just a little bruised, and very thirsty."

"Hold on."

Brax walked to the kitchen, found a pitcher of water and a cup, returned to her and said, "Here, drink."

He knew they should leave but he could see how dehydrated she was. She drank two cups of water. Lotus looked at Brax and saw true concern for her in his expression. She felt the impulse to tell him she loved him but had never said those words to him before, so instead she asked, "Brax, do you think you love me?"

Brax thought this was an odd time for such a question but knew she was overtaken with emotion after this harrowing experience, so he answered, "I don't have to think to breathe the air; neither do I have to think I love you. You are the air I breathe, and without you, I would suffocate."

Lotus's eyes welled with tears. She said "I love you too" and fell into his arms, exhausted.

"We must go now before anyone returns. But first, I am putting this man in the box you were in," Brax said. He did so, using the same rope and gag they had used on Lotus.

"They'll think the man left with me," said Lotus.

"Exactly," Brax replied. "Hopefully that will buy us some time."

They made their way back to the restaurant.

"How did you know I was there?" asked Lotus.

"I delivered a bag of grain to that cabin this morning. The bag busted open a little when I put it on the front porch of the cabin. I saw money mixed in with the grain. This told me where he was taking the money he collected. Then, on the path back to the restaurant, I found a scarf that looked like yours, and when I smelled the perfume on it, I *knew* it was yours. Since it wasn't far from the cabin, it only made sense that you were in there."

As they walked, Brax said, "Your grandmother said you had gone to your aunt's. I overheard them talking but Dakor pulled me away when I got there."

"He thinks my father told my grandmother where the emerald is so she could keep it safe in case something happened to him."

"I wouldn't have guessed she knew," said Brax.

"Me, neither," said Lotus.

"When I was listening in on Master Dakor's conversation, I did hear him say, "he intended to give her until noon on the second day to tell him where it is."

As they got close to the Cat's Claw, they came to a wild area with trees and large bushes. Brax said, "You can hide here. No one will be able to see you. I'll go ask your grandmother what she may have told Master Dakor before he left."

After he left for the delivery that morning, Master Dakor decided to apply more pressure to Tessa. He told her he had Lotus and that he knew Master Blade told her where the emerald is. He demanded that she tell him its location. When she refused, he took her by the shoulders, shook her, and yelled, "I know he told you!" She was terrified, but she thought quickly and tried to buy time, hoping a customer would come in, or that Master Blade would return early. She said, "He did not tell me where it is! But he did tell me that should something happen to him, I should go through his secret papers and the place he put it would be revealed there." She then told Master

270

Dakor that she would have the information ready for him when he returned.

"I will be back by noon on the second day," said Master Dakor.

"I will find out where it is and have Brax deliver it to you at that time, by the tree in the middle of the field across from the pond, on the old spice path just outside town," said Tessa. This was the same sugar maple tree Lotus and Brax sat beneath several days earlier.

"I will be passing by there exactly at noon. Be sure to have the emerald in hand. I will release Lotus after I have it," said Master Dakor. Tessa tearfully agreed.

After hearing about how Brax had handled the bandits he sent to kill him, Master Dakor was curious to know who he was, so he asked Tessa, "How did Brax end up working here? Where did Lotus find him?"

Not knowing it was a secret, Tessa told him something Lotus had said to her - that she had seen Brax come to the restaurant to retrieve a bag of grain for Master Talon before he worked there.

"I remembered that too," Tessa said. "I met him at the door that day. That's all I know."

Master Dakor got a look of fire in his eye. "Hmm, he is Master Talon's student. I will crush him and show him what real force is."

At that moment, Tessa realized she shouldn't have said anything about Brax.

As Master Dakor left, he said, "I'll be there at noon! Do not disappoint me!"

Master Dakor wanted to stay and make her go through the papers but had to leave because of his meeting. However, he wasn't worried because he thought he was holding all the cards. The special meeting was with his new, soon-to-be hired bandits. He needed a small group of fighters to help intimidate Master Blade by applying the cold force and disrupting his balance before he returned. He didn't want to miss that meeting because their leader was impatient and would leave if he was late.

When Brax returned to the restaurant, he saw Tessa with her head down, weeping at the back-corner table. He walked over to her. Before he could say anything, she raised her face and said, "I must tell you - Lotus did not go to her aunt's house. Master Dakor forced me to say that. But now, to make sure she is returned safely, I must give him the emerald. He told me he must have it on the second day at noon, when he returns with his men. I told him I would retrieve it and have you meet him at the tree in the field across from the pond."

Brax wanted to tell her right away that he had already rescued Lotus but was worried that if he did, she wouldn't give him the information he needed to protect them and himself from Master Dakor. All the attacks on him had started to make him distrustful too. At present, there were only two people in the world he trusted completely - Lotus and Master Talon.

"Lotus's tree?" he asked.

"Yes," said Tessa.

"Why there?"

"To buy time. The emerald is behind a stone in an opening under the tree. I needed time to come up with a solution, or in case Master Blade came back. He's due to arrive home next week. I hope he returns early. If so, no one would dare try to take the emerald. If he doesn't, you must get the emerald and give it to him to get my granddaughter back."

She seemed too sincere to be hiding anything. Unable to let her worry any longer, Brax said, "I rescued Lotus. She's hiding in the woods not far from here."

Tessa sighed with relief. "Oh, thank goodness. Is she okay?"

"Yes, she's fine. I still must meet Master Dakor or this will not stop. Somehow, I do not see him leaving if he gets the emerald," said Brax.

"I must tell you," Tessa said, "I didn't know I shouldn't have told him where I thought you worked before you came here. He knows now that you're Master Talon's student. He seemed determined to make an example of you. I am so sorry."

"Don't worry. Everything will be okay," said Brax. "I'm going to hide Lotus somewhere safe."

To protect Tessa, he didn't tell her or anyone else where he would hide Lotus, but he planned to take her to Master Talon. She would be safer with him than she would be anywhere else.

Meanwhile, a few towns over, Master Dakor bumped into an old bandit friend on his way to the next town meeting. They had lunch together and Master Dakor took the opportunity to add him to his growing gang of henchmen.

"Come work for me. I will have a lot of money soon, enough to raise a small army."

"How?" the bandit asked.

"I know where the Crown Prince Emerald is! It will be handed to me in two days."

"Interesting, If you have found the emerald, then the bigger prize must be near."

"What bigger prize?" asked Master Dakor.

"It is a prize worth much more. It is the crown prince's jewel."

"What is it?"

"It is a girl. It was said that she was hidden when the crown prince and his wife died, but most think she died at the same time," said the bandit.

"How do you know this?" asked Master Dakor.

"My drunkard uncle was their servant when I was young. I heard him tell this tale many times."

"How does this make her worth more than the emerald?" asked Master Dakor.

"The crown prince's evil sister is now ruling, but this girl is the rightful queen," said the bandit. "I am sure the current queen will want her silenced. I will definitely work for you now!"

"I have this girl held captive now," said Master Dakor. "Go tell the queen and ask her how much she would pay to get rid of her, never to be found."

"Okay. Make sure she is not hurt until we find out what the queen wants us to do."

"Fine, now go! I must leave to travel to the next town. You can meet me upon my return at the place where I will get the emerald. I will meet you there at noon in two days."

They both left.

Meanwhile, Brax walked back to get Lotus. It was very dark in the woods where she was hiding. As he got close, he whispered her name.

"I am here, Brax," she said.

Brax found her and took her hand to help her up. She hugged him tightly.

"Let's go under the camouflage of darkness. I am going to Master Talon to ask him to take care of you until I can sort this out. I'm sure he will agree. You will be safe there."

They made their way to Master Talon's shop. The pale moonlight was barely enough to light their way, but they still did their best to travel in the shadows, knowing any number of eyes could be concealed in the gloom of the forest surrounding them.

Jade Chi Do

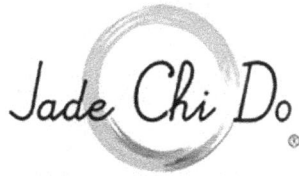

PART II - CHAPTER 19

Time to Rest

Brax and Lotus arrived at Master Talon's shop. Brax told him everything that had happened. "I was wondering if it would be okay if we . . ."

"Of course you can stay here," Master Talon interjected. "Let's sit and have some tea."

They walked to the back and joined him at a table in the sun. After so much time in the cold forest, they welcomed the warmth. Master Talon looked at both of them with compassion at first, but his eyes slowly became very serious as he looked right at Brax.

"Master Dakor will attempt to use your fear in a way that breaks your intention with the use of the warm force."

"How?" Brax asked.

"I see now that you love Lotus very much."

"Yes, I do, at a level I never thought possible," Brax replied.

"The key is the use of the warm force compared to the cold force use of love."

"I don't understand what you mean. How does this relate to my love for Lotus?"

"I will give you a more detailed explanation - because just as love can blind, it can also deafen, or more correctly, overwhelm one's hearing," Master Talon said with a smile.

He could see that Brax was still a little confused so he continued, "Let's trade places with one that would use the cold force to win. If you knew your opponent had the potential of being very powerful in directing warm life force, you would need to distract him to break the flow of his innermost intention directing the warm force. By doing this, it would provide a crack to enter and disrupt your balance. Once one is off balance, immediate and relentless effort would be made to achieve victory."

"Okay, I understand that, but how could he do this to me?" Brax asked.

"By overwhelming you with fear by implanting the image in your mind of losing Lotus. He will use against you that which you love most."

Brax thought for a moment, then looked down and said, "I see now. This is truly my weakness."

"Brax, I'm going to give you the key now that will give you strength and more focused attention. Are you ready?"

"Yes," Brax replied eagerly.

"The key is to love Lotus."

"I do love her, but you said my love is my weakness," Brax replied.

"No, Brax. The key is not to stop loving, even if such a thing were possible, it is to go further into your love and trust that unconditional love connects us all. Your love of Lotus must rise like a true lotus flower, emerging victoriously from the swamp and muck of this world. See your love of Lotus as perfect and beautiful, unbroken, indestructible. When fear of the loss of love happens, is it not you - your ego - that is worried you may lose her? Instead, allow her love to empower you to direct the warm force. Know that her love is aligned and connected with you from deep within. Raw, pure love is the energy that binds the warm force of life."

Brax meditated on this for a long moment and the wisdom of it connected within him as surely as the sprockets of a clock locking into place.

"I understand. Aligning our love as one empowers the connection to the warm force." Brax thought a little more and said, "I feel I am prepared. I am seeing and connecting more of your lessons. I see how Master Dakor uses the cold force to pull fear out of the shopkeepers. By giving them a sense of potential loss, he creates a crack to bend their needs to his will."

"Good point, Brax. A defense here would be like water, as water will remove rock over time, yet remain water. Water and the warm life force are similar because water remains whole. One. Even if separated, it may move to a different form, but it does not change. Using water as an example, the shopkeepers can help themselves by resolving to only acquiesce to Master Dakor's demands in the short term. In the meantime, seek to align with those that do not give in, in many numbers. In time, this will overcome and be victorious."

"Sadly, from what I've seen, most just keep swimming in fear perpetually and give its flow of cold force to Master Dakor," Brax said.

Brax and Lotus spent the day together. When it was starting to get dark, Brax found Master Talon because he wanted to ask him something he was curious about. He was standing in the kitchen, making dinner.

"Ah, just in time, lovebirds! I think you'll enjoy this. Old family recipe."

"It smells delicious," Lotus said.

"Sure does!" Brax added.

"Have a seat there. It's almost finished," Master Talon said, smiling over his shoulder.

When he had set the dinner out and joined them, Brax said, "Master Talon, may I ask - why do you not fight in combat?"

"Nothing like a little light conversation over dinner. Eh, Lotus?" Master Talon joked. Lotus giggled.

"I'm sorry . . . I -"

"It's okay, Brax. I was wondering when you would ask that. The most obvious answer is that I am very old, but this is not the main reason. It is because I have made a choice to no longer play with the cold force and its deceptions. I know there is a place for this in battle, sport, and even business. It is part of this world. It exists around those who play and feed on the cold force. But with teachers like me, the use of the cold force could do more harm. The fact is, you do not become bad when you use the cold force, but of those who use it out of necessity, it is inevitable that some of them will continue beyond necessity, feeding and controlling others with fear, doubt, and uncertainty. I have laid my sword down, but I do teach because without one teaching the use of the warm force of chi, the cold force would be the only known way to achieve such connection, giving greater possibility of more chaos and unrest in the world by those who feed on others as sheep. Until my last breath, I will teach the use of the warm force as a home to settle in versus the illusion of security in the cold force. I am humbled by the opportunity to help others find that which is within them that lays waiting to be discovered. In your case, I am glad that you have been so diligent and have progressed so well because it is inevitable that Master Dakor will challenge you to an Earthen Palm match. Be sure to review your lesson on this." *

Brax promised he would and thanked Master Talon for the explanation, then they retired for the evening. As they relaxed in the bedroom, Lotus said, "Brax, I'm confused about something. When I

281

was watching Master Talon train you earlier, when you were both facing each other at the table, you seemed to be listening to him very intently even when he was saying very little, or even not talking at all. It was as if you were hearing something I didn't. You would respond to him for several minutes after I had only heard him say a few words. I can't explain it."

Brax was baffled. "I'm not sure what happened. This is the first time I have had anyone watch me learn from Master Talon. I heard him talking the whole time. This is a surprise to me. Whatever you were experiencing, I was unaware of it. I just assumed you could hear him too. I will ask him about it."

Brax noticed a flicker of light from the window. He looked out and saw Master Talon sitting by a firepit in the back. It was a circle of stones with wooden benches around it.

"Let's go sit by the campfire," Brax suggested to Lotus.

"Sounds good to me."

They walked out and sat on one of the benches.

"Good evening, Master Talon," said Brax.

"Good evening to you both," said Master Talon.

"The fire feels nice. It's very cool tonight," said Lotus.

"Yes, it is. Thank you for joining me."

"It is our honor, and thank you," said Lotus.

As they enjoyed the fire, light breezes moved the smoke in various directions. As Brax watched, something caught his attention. When the smoke blew toward Master Talon, he would lift his right hand at the wrist and hold it up a little, seemingly diverting the smoke around and away from him. He did not say anything, but looked forward to learning this from him someday too. Being young, Brax thought of it as merely a cool trick, but he was mature enough to know it was much more than that.

Master Talon said, "I'm going to find more firewood. I'll be right back."

Brax looked at Lotus staring into the blue flames, lost in thought, and whispered, "What are you thinking about?"

"It's more like what I'm trying *not* to think about - your meeting with Master Dakor tomorrow. I worry for your safety. I love you so much."

Brax put his arm around her and pulled her close. When he said "I love you too", his mind immediately traveled back to the lesson Master Talon had taught him about being prepared for Master Dakor to use his love against him. He wondered how somebody could become so corrupted, so lustful for power that they would abuse love - the most sacred emotion human beings can feel. It not only confused him, it angered him as well, another emotion that masters of the cold force like Master Dakor could use against him.

Brax lifted and lightly kissed the back of her hand, then held her soft hand to his cheek. "Don't worry. No matter what happens, I know

now our love will be our strength, not something he can use to weaken us."

As he lifted his face to look at her, she noticed the fire's reflection flickering in his eyes and thought she could stay in this moment forever.

"Brax, we can just run away," said Lotus.

"I don't think that would stop him. Your father would be taken by surprise because only I know what Dakor's planning - recruiting a gang of men to take over the restaurant and use it as his base of operations. The emerald will give him the extra money he needs to expand his plans."

Lotus said sadly, "I understand. You're right. We can't run from this." She looked at Brax with fear in her eyes.

"Everything will be okay. Don't worry," Brax said.

Lotus smiled and said, "Okay. I'm going in to get ready for bed."

"I'll join you in a little while. I need to talk with Master Talon some more."

She kissed him on the cheek. As she walked toward their room, she passed Master Talon carrying firewood back to the firepit.

"Goodnight, Master Talon. Thank you again for letting us stay here."

"You're welcome. Rest well."

Brax and Master Talon sat gazing into the fire. Brax broke the silence.

"This may not be the place, but may I ask you one more question?" Brax laughed, anticipating that he would give his usual response of "You just asked me one question."

Master Talon knew why he was laughing and started laughing too. Finally, he said, "Okay, I won't say it again. What is it that you want to ask?"

"Lotus asked me about something I never noticed before. When you were teaching me, she said you were saying less words audibly than I was hearing from you. I know this sounds strange. She said she could not hear everything you were saying so the lesson didn't make complete sense to her."

"Brax, this is a complicated subject. We have much to talk about. In many ways, you are ready to be able to learn more. I will teach you in a way that will allow you to grow tangibly. I could explain this to you, but as always, it is best you learn more first and grow into this knowledge. Experience is always superior to listening to speeches. But I will give you an example. When a tree starts growing, its roots reach out in many directions to stabilize the tree, but the tree needs to grow first. Roots are like your lessons - reinforced by dedication and continued repetition. It then will express itself in tangible fruits. We must address this further as you grow. But I will say, a teacher will talk with fewer words as you progress and develop a stronger vocabulary regarding what one word or a group of words mean. As the student receives compounded information based on prior lessons, less and less is said by the teacher to convey a larger lesson and meaning."

He paused for a minute, not wanting to overwhelm Brax, but he did need to share more, so he added, "When one has a unique focus, one can convey much to the person listening, especially when their inner attention is focused on it. To a person watching, it will seem that few words are said. This may be confusing but it will make more sense as you grow. You have just reached the tangible elevation in your training. This enables you to go forward to your next elevation and create palpable benefits from this."

Brax nodded in agreement and said, "I understand that *tangible* means the senses and peaked abilities that can be felt within myself and in the world around me."

"You have a good start on understanding your growth with the training and lessons to come," said Master Talon happily. "Before I put this fire out and we all retire for the evening, I have a lesson for you. You are welcome to share this lesson with your future children."

Brax said, "Of course. Please do!"

Master Talon bringing up the idea of future children got him a little excited and curious. Master Talon smiled as if recalling some happy memory and said, "This is a lesson I taught to my most precious son. He was young and he would argue with his mother a lot. One day I arrived home to find that he was sent to his room. He was not happy. I went in to talk to him. My heart felt for him, he was so angry. I asked him, 'Can you get a piece of paper and draw something for me?' He did.

"I said, 'Please draw me a picture of two fires across from each other.' He did that too."

"Then I asked him, 'What would happen if the two fires got together?'"

"He said, 'Dad, that's a no brainer - a bigger fire!'"

"I said, 'Okay, now would you say fire is like anger?'"

"He answered, 'Of course, Dad!'"

"Then I said, 'Now draw me a bucket of water on the same paper.'"

"He agreed, then drew a bucket with lines looking like water."

"I said, 'Son, if you poured water on the fire, what would happen?'"

"He said, 'It would put it out.'"

"I said, 'Okay, Son, then who was the winner? Water or fire?'"

"He said, 'Water!'"

"I then asked, 'Do you want to be the winner or the fire?'"

"He looked as if a light went off in his mind, then he said, 'It is water, for sure!'"

I said, 'Son, as you agreed, two fires turn into a bigger fire. It also always needs more fuel to keep it burning, so one ends up always looking for fuel to feed the fire. Our anger, just like a campfire, needs wood - fuel - to keep burning. Water is the victor. Be the winner.'"

"After this, my son chose to be the winner most times, and he turned out to be an awesome father himself," Master Talon said proudly as Brax gazed at the campfire.

"I will never look at another campfire the same way again," Brax said. "Thank you for sharing your personal life with me. I am honored."

Master Talon picked up a bucket of water and put the fire out.

Laughing a little, Brax said, "And the water just won!"

They walked back to go to sleep.

"See you in the morning, Brax. Sleep well."

"Goodnight, Master."

* Reference chapter 16

Jade Chi Do

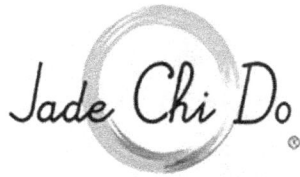

PART II - CHAPTER 20

A Zone Away

As Brax, Lotus, and Master Talon ate breakfast the next morning, Brax said, "I think I should go to work so I don't raise any suspicion."

"That is a good idea," said Master Talon.

"I agree," Lotus said. "My grandmother has been taking my place at the restaurant a lot lately. It would be good if you helped her. Please tell her I'm okay."

"Brax, I am going to give you a quick lesson this morning so you can get there earlier," Master Talon said.

"Oh?" Brax replied.

"Can I join the training today?" Lotus asked. "I would like to start learning this art from you."

This surprised Brax and he was about to say it was not a good idea because he thought Master Talon would have some intense special training planned in preparation for his meeting with Master Dakor the next day, but as soon as he started to speak, Master Talon said, "Yes, today's training lesson is a perfect fit. It is best to go back to the beginning training of our art before a possible challenge like Brax has tomorrow. Having confidence in everything you've trained so far - your foundation - will stand by you in the heat of battle. But remember, when a challenge comes your way, do not let your confidence be destroyed. Now if you will come with me."

Master Talon led them to the rear training area and said, "Sit in the chairs behind you, facing me."

They both sat. Brax was a little distracted with Lotus there. He found himself looking at her. Master Talon noticed and said, "Look forward." They both did so.

"This lesson involves the speed of the body. Your breath pattern of nose or mouth, chest or belly is not a concern with today's lesson. But when you practice more, inhale into your belly with your nose, and exhale with your mouth. Okay, let's start. This lesson is called **Distance Zones**. First, close your eyes and start following your breath. Say to yourself as you keep your posture aligned, "I am like a tree, observing but not thinking." A tree does not think like we do. See yourself as the tree, feeling the wind, oblivious to yesterday or tomorrow, aware only of the moment the wind hits it," said Master Talon.

Lotus was amazed at how much simply seeing herself as the tree calmed her.

"Next, lay your hands on each thigh, above the knees. Keep your palms facing up toward the sky. Open your hands, starting with your fingers. It is important that you breathe in as you slowly open your hands."

Master Talon then said, "Lotus, imagine you're breathing in through your hands as you slowly open them. Next, as you breathe out, slowly close your hands and imagine your breath leaving your palms. Keep repeating this exercise as you breathe."

He already knew Brax could feel the warm force and direct it with or without his breath, so he added a little more instruction for Lotus to get her started. After a few minutes of both of them doing this exercise, he said, "I want you to keep doing this, and I will teach you an additional exercise to add to it. Do both of these exercises at the same time."

They both kept doing the exercise as Master Talon added the additional parts.

"Next, while your eyes are still closed, visualize your leg extending to kick an opponent. Next, visualize seeing your foot extended outward and where the line would stop if your foot was extended as far as it can go. Now imagine the farthest your leg would extend. Visualize this now as a circle around you. This is called the leg zone. Next, extend your arm out and visualize the maximum distance. Imagine a line at this distance all around you. This is called your arm zone. Next is your elbow zone. Repeat the same process, visualize it extended, then visualize the closer line all around you. Once you have completed each step, visualize looking down and around you, imagining all three circles. Breathe your intention to be aware of this. This ties into our physical awareness. Being sensitive to these three distances will help improve your awareness."

As Brax and Lotus practiced this, he continued, "In general combat, a leg zone is good for keeping an opponent at a distance, but is slower to defend then the faster hand/arm zone. The elbow zone is very fast, yet loss of distance can create much confusion. Many weapons are used in the elbow zone. The fourth zone is your body zone. When an attack goes there, it goes to a ground fight in many cases. This body zone should be avoided because if you're on the ground, others may attack you. The body zone is good for sport as you do not have two or more potential attackers hitting you while you fight. However, it is important to learn all zones as you may only be in combat with one person. I am not teaching you here how to use your training, but to open your awareness and connect the warm force to it. A simple expression would be to back you up, with the higher goal of seeing attacks at their inception. This can also benefit someone in business, sports, and many other professions. Connecting these visualization exercises to the palm breathing exercise of the warm force will increase the abilities within you."

"Remember," Master Talon added, "when you connect with your inner, serving self, it looks out for you in a small, almost inaudible voice. For instance, you can randomly read something - a newspaper or a page from a book chosen seemingly at random - and later find out that there was a message woven into it that helped you on the path you have been searching for, sometimes not even consciously knowing you were. This art of Jade Chi Do is to create a clear path to this, while also lowering your personal blinders so you can hear, connect, and communicate with the inner self that is there for you and always has been. With further practice, you will discover further abilities with use of the warm force. Its expression will be exponentially expressed in all you do as you expand your personal paradigm."

He then looked at Lotus and said, "Okay, Lotus. This will conclude your training with Brax today. I have a couple more lessons to add to this for him."

"Thank you for giving me a lesson today," Lotus said.

Brax turned and smiled.

"You're welcome," Master Talon said.

Lotus went to the bedroom to freshen up as Brax and Master Talon continued training.

Master Talon said, "I have taught this to you today to relay a couple of deeper lessons. You may recognize similar references to zones in combat arts. The difference is that I intertwined this in a recipe for this lesson today to increase a greater outcome and growth within you. As always, to fully understand and apply this teaching, you must go beyond the assumptions you might make based upon your prior training. Confirmations of prior interpretations can deafen you to new discoveries. A way to get around this habit is to tell yourself, 'Just for a moment, I will imagine that this lesson, or this part of the lesson, is completely new to me.' In other words, truly be an empty cup. Empty your mind so it can be filled again without overflowing. Would it be easier for you to see this and learn it?"

"I think so," Brax replied, feeling more awakened. "Even though I feel I know this, hearing this from you truly brings it into perspective. Thank you. I have a wealth of training and it has helped me a lot, but the flip side of it is it may limit my ability to expand upon it. If I am honest with myself, I feel perhaps it's a sort of fear, in a way, or my ego; a fear of losing the identity of the fighting style I learned, especially through repetition. But in fact, I must let go to gain more!"

"I couldn't have said it better myself," said Master Talon. He paused for a few seconds, looking at Brax. "You understand well, but it goes even deeper than that. Allow me to share something with you that will show you where your mind is at. I will teach you an exercise to practice, and a way to increase your perception. First, your exercise - as you walk to work today, walk with the meditation I taught you where you see all around yourself." *

Brax immediately remembered this walking training that helped him achieve a special experience momentarily, but then he lost it because he got excited. *

Master Talon continued, "Now, with this exercise in mind, add to your inner intentions, imagining these four zones. Envision them in your imagination as circles around your back and front; a complete circle. As you walk, recognize these distance point zones from today's lesson. Walk as if the circles are there, always around you. This will communicate something very special to yourself, and it will affect

294

your expression of your awareness in a very special way. With practice, you will discover great abilities in this that have been waiting within you all along. I do not call it evolution, just discovery of what has always been there, waiting for you to find and use it. This is why I have hastened this within you. I feel this practice will be condensed and will even help you tomorrow. I am happy you continued to practice your training from the beginning. That will enable you to continue to excel and properly digest later lessons so they too can become tangible. Be sure to practice today."

"I will," Brax replied eagerly. He felt a little overwhelmed with the confrontation looming the next day. He could tell Master Talon was filling him with new information to learn and exercises to practice so he would have very little room in his mind to think about it and worry. He also understood why Master Talon chose such a different training today. He trusted the process, and was excited to work this in with the waking exercise he learned from his prior lessons. *

Master Talon continued, "Next, let's talk about perception. In this lesson, I will be talking directly to that person inside of you; that part of you that digests your lesson, and reviews them on the chalkboard of your dreams. Because you are truly growing with this art and adjusting to the benefits of being a practitioner of Jade Chi Do, it will reveal itself to you and you will be rewarded in all your professions. But for now, I will speak about combat. I will bring something to your attention that will help you grow, push through some illusionary walls holding you back, and increase the expressions of your abilities to react. Say your combat style reacts to an attack with a trained move to deactivate the offense. You will start from the point you trained from to achieve this. But due to your also being a practitioner of Jade Chi Do, you will see many attacks at their inception, all the way down to recognizing intention and opposing them - whether in a street fight, on the mat, or in business. Now, if your combat training only reacts to a strike to divert it, you may still wait for it to extend in that distance zone of comfort from your repetitive training."

"Repetitive?" asked Brax.

"Yes. As you know, our body as a whole learns moves by repetition to enter our reflexive mind. But in a deeper sense, through repetitive reactions to an attack, either in your imagination or physically, your body learns economy of motion, providing ease of speed."

"Okay, I understand this more now," said Brax.

"Good. To return to my next point, if you do not train further this way, to react to the inception of the attack, you will not do as well as you could. Most will let the ego decide, but I feel you will react well, as I will continue to share with you my knowledge dealing with the inception, and will amplify this by giving you your lesson with fewer words to hasten your progress."

Brax immediately remembered his conversation about this from his earlier question about what Lotus heard, or didn't hear, when Master Talon was talking to him, so he knew what he meant. Brax nodded and said, "I will do as you instructed and practice the distance zone, as in the walking meditation you taught me." *

Master Talon nodded his head in silent agreement, then they finished training and Master Talon said, "Brax, I know you are concerned about what is coming. Listen well. If you have to be in the storm, in the tornado of challenges, then be the eye of the storm. This is the calm place of leaders, giving them clarity within the storm. You've got this! Be the eye of the storm, not just another piece of debris sucked into the whirlwind and tossed about aimlessly, and you will be victorious. Trust the unity and power of how Jade Chi Do intertwines naturally with your prior learning. There are also your actions outside of the calm. You are also the one reacting to an attack. You are the center of the fight. Everyone else is attacking into the center, as if charging toward a tornado only to bounce off it because of its impenetrable strength. In this light, you are also the storm, reacting from the calm."

Finally, Master Talon said, "Brax, I know you must get going to work. Remember that Lotus has chosen to learn Jade Chi Do as well, so you will have a great partner to work the exercises with, and this will amplify your growth."

Brax smiled and thanked him, then kissed Lotus goodbye and left for work.

"I will see you later," Lotus said confidently.

As Brax walked away, he replied, "I will keep seeing you in my mind always."

"Please be careful and don't forget to tell my grandmother I'm okay."

"I will," Brax promised.

She watched Brax walk away until she couldn't see him anymore. Master Talon could tell she was worried. "Come. Let's have some tea," he said.

When Brax arrived at the Cat's Claw restaurant, Lotus's grandmother met him at the front door.

"Hello, Brax. I've been waiting for you. Is Lotus okay?"

"Yes, she is good and well," said Brax.

"I am glad you arrived early, before it got busy. I have more to tell you."

They both walked over to a corner table, away from the kitchen. "I must tell you a secret about Lotus. This will possibly make things much worse if Master Dakor finds out. Lotus is the crown prince's daughter."

"That is a surprise, but how does it matter?" asked Brax.

"It is because she is the rightful heir to the throne. The crown prince's evil sister has taken the throne, and there is a widespread rumor that she had him and his family killed to do so. But Master Blade was able to save the child - Lotus - and with his dying breath, the crown prince gave the emerald and care of Lotus to Master Blade . . . my son, his most trusted warrior. As you know now, he raised her as his own."

"I did not know this. You're right - if he learns this, Lotus is in more danger," Brax said, more worried than ever.

"If Master Blade returns, I will send him out to where the meeting will be," Tessa decided.

"Thank you. I must start work now," Brax said. He walked to the kitchen.

It was a busy day, and the help Master Dakor hired did not show up. Tessa and Brax were overwhelmed but he was thankful it was busy because it made the day go by quickly. He could not wait to get back to Lotus.

The day ended late and he made his way back to Master Talon's shop. He practiced the day's lesson in near darkness but found it intensified the lesson tremendously. He was happy Master Talon gave him this lesson for more than one reason, the main one being it filled his mind so much, the doubt of the cold force could not weaken him.

* Reference Chapter 8.

Jade Chi Do

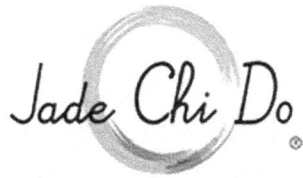

PART II - CHAPTER 21

Meeting at the Tree

W hen Brax arrived at Master Talon's Shop, everyone was asleep so he made his way to the bedroom and fell fast asleep. He awoke early the next morning and met Master Talon to see if he wanted to give him any additional training before he left for the restaurant.

"You have a big day ahead of you," Master Talon said. "This morning, we will fill your thoughts with perspective and your inner self will tie much together for you. Don't try to memorize; just trust that part of you will be listening. This will indeed help you. Where there is confidence that is unable to be broken, there is the seed for success. You may have seen in some sports, when it appears that one team is doomed, the other team comes through in the end, with only seconds left on the clock, and emerges victorious."

"Yes, I have noticed this," said Brax.

"Brax, our training has helped you gain the ability to see movements at their inception and accelerate your reaction time to external incoming actions. Today, we will include the internal in the same fashion. I'm going to teach you this because you will need this perspective if you get hurt. In combat, there are also distractions from within. We have talked about how Master Dakor may use the cold force by using your love for Lotus to distract you.

But in case he causes you physical pain in some way, either by his touch, striking past your body, or attacking a vital point on a limb, what I'm going to go over with you in more depth is this - in any conflict, one must stop and direct the train - the path - of pain or fear to continue to engage at an optimal level. Meditate on these thoughts so that this concept may unfold within you."

"It may weaken you and add to your challenges if fear and pain are allowed free reign. Think of it this way - when a cup of water is tipped and starts to fall, when would be the best time to stop the water from spilling?"

Brax replied, "It would be before the water starts to pour out, of course. But if I did not know when it would start due to someone bumping it, for example, or some unrelated choice - that is, if it were someone else's choice to tip it over - I could only react to the act once the choice was made to drop or tip the cup. In this case, to hold the most water in, I would need to catch the cup as quickly as I could when it started to fall."

"Correct. Fear and pain from within are no different. They are both messengers. If we ignore them, they will turn up their trumpet, or volume, louder until you cannot move. So face the fear. In addition to being a messenger, pain can merely be fear as well. Now let me ask you another question. What is one gift we are all given that the cold force wants us to give away?"

"The ability to choose," Brax replied.

"Right again. One thing that we have on this earth is choice. If we make a bad choice, we pay for it one way or another. We can learn from it and make better choices, and we can learn from others as well. I have provided something to you that gives you more to choose from to go further within yourself, but the choice is always yours. Now, I would like to explore inner pain and fear further because giving you a strong, internal perspective will reward you with the least amount of effort. For example, in some cases, extremely cold weather will freeze one person but not another. Would you agree it is at inception - the very beginning - that either person will interpret the action occurring to them?"

"Yes," Brax affirmed.

"Likewise, if a sled is about to slide down a hill and you want to stop it before it hurts someone, what is the best time to do this?"

"At the very start, or at best, before it gains momentum, the same as with the physical action," said Brax.

"You're right. It is the same with a physical or internal attack, or even a cold temperature trying to radiate into your body. Whether an internal and external force like a punch, verbal attack, cold weather, etcetera, changing one's perception or interpretation at its inception will create higher and longer tolerance, stretching the paradigm beyond what we thought possible."

"I see," Brax answered.

"Good. Before you leave, meditate as a tree just to clear your mind."

"To be sure I understand correctly, this meditation is where we start, but depending on the lesson, we go further?" Brax suggested.

"Yes, I teach you this lesson today knowing the part of you that is there to serve you is listening. Have this confidence and all will be applied to whatever you're going to do. In this case, it is not business or sport, but the coming combat. There are many meditations, and as you know, many are interconnected. For our purposes, most different types of meditation are good and useful. In our training, meditation is not just a way of taking a vacation or communing with your pure consciousness, though there are times when that is useful too. As you know from your prior training, we seek to interact with this world as well, evolving, or more accurately, discovering that which already lays waiting within us, expanding our paradigm."

They sat and meditated silently for a while. Brax closed his eyes, feeling the wind against his face, tossing his hair, enjoying this moment of peace before the troublesome events of the day ahead.

"Brax, we are done today. You are ready," Master Talon said.

Lotus walked over to Brax and hugged him tightly. "Please be careful. Should I go with you?" she asked.

"No. Thank you, but it is safer to stay with Master Talon."

Brax left to go to the meeting place. Meanwhile, Master Dakor was on his way, two towns away, returning from his dark business. The bandit, Robdo, the one he sent to meet the evil queen, had returned earlier and met Master Dakor at the town where they first met.

"Master Dakor," Robdo said. "I met with Queen Teraw. She received your message about Lotus. I hurried back to relay her conditions to you. She will reward you with your weight in gold if you secretly deliver Lotus to her alive and unharmed. She will offer additional rewards for other wanted bounties to retrieve for her. All conditions must be met. She also said you would be rewarded further based on how fast you get this done."

"I am surprised that delivering her head would not be enough," replied Master Dakor.

"Their must be a bigger plan," Robdo said.

Master Dakor thought for a moment and said, "Thank you for this information. I have only received half of the men I was going to get. I was told at my meeting the rest are away on another job and they will be back in a week. I have nine, including you. I must change my plans. I will get Lotus at the cabin and deliver her to queen Teraw. Take four men and go to the tree meeting. Get there early to destroy Brax and retrieve the emerald."

Master Dakor did not know this, but the queen knew that if Lotus were alive, she could leverage this against Master Blade, for if the rumors were true, the crown prince would have shared with him where he hid many other valuable items and information. Acquiring such treasures and knowledge would intensify her power over her people.

The bandit, Robdo, did as he was asked. The five bandits, including himself, left as fast as they could to the meeting spot at the tree. They arrived earlier than Brax. Robdo told three of his men to stay hidden and watch for Brax. He said, "If anyone comes with Brax, be ready to attack them."

Meanwhile, Lotus was so stricken with worry, she snuck away from Master Talon's shop and followed the path she thought Brax would take in hopes of helping him in some way. Brax did not know this, and he was about twenty minutes ahead of her. As he was walking to the tree, he thought Master Dakor would probably challenge him to an earthen palm match, as Master Talon had predicted. He thought Master Dakor would make a bet that if he fell first, he would leave and never return, and if Brax lost, he would give him the Crown Prince Emerald. Going with the challenge was better than having to fight master Dakor and all his men. He thought this may be his best shot for a more peaceful solution.

When Brax arrived, he could see two men standing by the tree. As he got closer, he said, "Where is Master Dakor? He is supposed to meet me here."

"No. The plans have changed," Robdo said. "Where is the emerald?"

"You are not going to get it," Brax said sternly.

The two men looked at each other. Enraged, they attacked Brax, but he easily defended himself. He had just finished with them when he heard a scream. He looked and saw the three men who were hiding. They had Lotus. Brax was shocked, which gave one of the bandits the opportunity to attack. He hit Brax hard in the chest. Brax fell and was standing back up when Robdo yelled, "They will hurt her if you do not give us the emerald!"

Brax thought for a moment and said, "Bring her closer to me so I can see she's alright, then I will give you the emerald."

Robdo had no fear because the other four men were there to back him up. He nodded to the three bandits to bring Lotus to Brax. They stood her next to him while one of them held her other arm.

"Okay, look at her," said Robdo.

Just then, Lotus turned and kicked the bandit who was holding her arm in the groin. He let go and dropped to his knees. She quickly stood behind Brax. The other men came at Brax. He moved instinctively and all became slow motion, as it did in his training. As they attacked him from all sides, he deactivated the attacks with strikes that were so severe, they were disabled in seconds and scattered on the ground, utterly defeated.

Lotus said, "Brax, that was incredible. Just as they started to move, you interrupted every attack with strikes that just devastated them. I have never seen you react like this. It was like you were flowing, in constant motion."

"Did they hurt you?" asked Brax.

"No. They seemed to be very careful *not* to hurt me," said Lotus with growing curiosity.

"Master Dakor must have gone to get you at the cabin."

"Yes, I fear that once he figures out I am not there, he will hurt my grandmother," said Lotus, fear rising in her voice.

"I must go and stop this."

"I'm going too!"

Brax looked at her, disappointed, knowing she didn't listen to him earlier, and said, "Let's go, but I will leave you with your grandmother."

They both left for the restaurant.

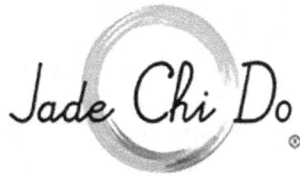

PART II - CHAPTER 22

Earthen Palm

"I worry about your safety," Brax said as he walked with Lotus.

"I don't want to leave your side, but I'll stay with my grandmother. She said my father is due back anytime."

"I remember when we first met, as I watched you cast the net into the water, you were so radiant. Who would have known it would have brought us to where we are now?" Brax said with a warm tone and love in his eyes.

"I love you too," she said, looking into his eyes. They hugged tightly, eyes closed, uncertainty about the future causing them to savor the peace they felt in each other's arms even more than usual.

On their way to the restaurant, just before town, there was a bridge over the river that supplied the mill. The river was fed by a waterfall further up. They had almost reached this bridge when, without warning, Master Dakor's men popped out of the wood line, grabbing Lotus. At the same time, Master Dakor yelled, "Do not fight, Brax, or she will be dead!" It was a bluff because to collect the bounty from the queen, he needed to take Lotus back to her alive and unharmed.

Brax stood still. His awareness was on Lotus when this happened. Angry with himself, he thought, *I should have felt this and not allowed myself to get distracted.*

Master Dakor walked out of the wood line into the field near the bridge and yelled to the bandit, "Bring her here! Bare her shoulder!"

The bandit did so, exposing the mark on her skin.

"Yes, it is the crown prince's crest," said Master Dakor. "We definitely have the right girl. Now, Brax, you will die."

Knowing Dakor had a big ego and loved to feed it, Brax replied, "I challenge you to an earthen palm match. The victor departs with Lotus. Or are you afraid?"

Master Dakor felt boxed in by the cold force that raged within him. He thought about this for a moment and almost said no since he already had the upper hand, but then he saw the faces of his thugs and knew they would lose respect for him if he backed down. Word might even get out that he cowered, so he yelled, "I accept, and you will regret it!"

His men stood around him, ready to pounce on Brax should anything go wrong for Master Dakor. They stood in front of each other. Brax bowed to signal the beginning, expecting Master Dakor to bow back, as was customary, but he only yelled, "I do not bow to the trash of Master Talon. Let's get on with this!"

They both got into the earthen palm stance, then put their right palms against each other, with their arms bent. Master Dakor said to one of the bandits, "Wait for a few minutes as we move back and forth to feel each other's chi, then shout 'Go!'"

As they stared, Master Talon's voice rang in Brax's mind . . . "You are in this moment. Let nothing distract you. Give your full, deep, innermost intention to deliver and direct the warm life force. Allow your vision to see and feel all his moves at their inception. Actively react, always feeling *I am the calm eye of the storm.* * Just then, all became slow motion, as if time did not exist.

"Go!" yelled the bandit.

An electrical charge as strong as a lightning bolt surged from Master Dakor's hand, carrying and passing more than just physical energy. Brax's elbow and shoulder absorbed it, then it dropped into his feet and dissipated into the earth.

Master Dakor gave Brax a look of worried surprise. Brax saw this and instinctively felt a weakness form in him, like hardened earth cracking open. He then sent the warm force from his feet all the way up through his hand. It had the same effect, as if a bolt of lightning went through Master Dakor. His knees buckled and he almost fell, but he quickly reacted and stood back up. He looked Brax in the eyes, and in an attempt to put a crack in Brax's use of the warm force, inflict injury, and get him to fall to the ground, he said, "Should I fall, I never said I would not make her suffer first, and I will enjoy it!"

It had the desired effect - Brax started to fall out of the zone. For a second or two, things were at regular speed and he could barely stay on his feet. But again, he heard Master Talon's voice . . . "Do not fear a loss that has not happened yet. Your love will be your strength."

Just then, he felt Master Dakor get ready to discharge his chi like before, but at the very start, Brax caught it and the physical force and energy traveling up from Master Dakor's foot only reached his shoulder. Brax stopped it at that location, dislocating his shoulder with a dull crack. Master Dakor dropped to the ground. Brax stood watching as Master Dakor got up and one of his bandits popped his shoulder back in.

"I have won. Now honor our agreement!" Brax demanded.

"Oh, I will, after I kill you." Master Dakor winced with pain, motioned to his bandits, and yelled, "Get him!"

They all started to stalk toward Brax except the one holding Lotus. All of a sudden, a thundering sound came from the woods, distracting them. As they looked over, Lotus's father, Master Blade, exploded out of the trees and quickly took out the man holding his daughter. He fell to the ground instantly. The other bandits saw this and attacked him. As he fought with them, Master Dakor looked at Brax and hissed, "Now I will destroy you."

Brax recognized that he was trying to push the fear of the cold force into him. The energy felt like a cold wind. He identified it quickly now that he was familiar with how the warm force felt. He thought, *This is the difference.* He felt his body react with warmth - a radiating of warm life force, shining like the sun, derailing Master Dakor's efforts.

They fought using their martial arts, then went back and forth, each reacting at the inception of each movement. They moved with great speed, yet each only saw each other moving in slow motion. One of the bandits, badly beaten by Master Blade, grabbed Lotus and started backing up with her, using her as a shield to get away. Brax heard her scream, and in that second, he disconnected from his intention. Master Dakor sensed this crack and struck quickly. Brax fell to the ground. Master Dakor leaned over him to give the final death strike as Brax struggled to recover fast enough to defend himself, but his love for Lotus and fear of losing her streamed into his heart. As Brax looked up, he saw a flash of white light and started to see in slow motion again. He then saw Master Talon move in between them, come closer, and look into Brax's eyes. His eyes were full of white fire. Brax felt cold chills race through him.

In a split second, Brax watched Master Talon, still looking at him, raise his right elbow behind him, swing his palm out, and strike Master Dakor's chest. It was so fast, Master Dakor still had his hand held up to strike Brax. There was a sound like a tree snapping or a thick board breaking. Lotus and the bandit watched as Master Dakor's ribs and spine were blown outward, the jagged edges of the fractured bones splitting the skin and protruding from his back. Master Dakor dropped without taking another breath.

Brax laid there with an injured chest, struggling to breathe. Master Talon placed his hand on his chest. Brax felt a sharp wave of warmth, and with it, an overwhelming feeling of love and concern for Lotus filled his chest. Suddenly, he could breathe much easier again. He stood up and looked at the remaining bandits. They scrambled to their feet and ran away.

Master Blade ran to Lotus to make sure she was okay. Brax was standing next to her.

"Father, this is Brax," she said.

"Thank you for all you have done," Master Blade said.

Brax looked at Master Talon. "Thank you for saving my life."

"I must tell you something," Master Talon replied. "When Dakor killed my teacher, I wanted to get revenge. I found my teacher on the ground all alone, clinging to life. I felt the cold force run through my veins. I wanted to kill him, and would have, but with his last breath, my teacher made me promise not to seek revenge. He told me there would be a time when it would be right and that I would know when that time comes. He said the warm force would be at my side, and that I would direct warm and cold together. Only then would Dakor's time pass. That moment just arrived. I could not let him do this to you. Brax, you have taught me the completion of my teacher's last lesson. Thank you from the bottom of my heart," Master Talon said with tears in his eyes.

Then her father looked at Lotus and said, "Your journey has just begun. Now that these evil men know you're alive, many more will come. We should travel to get more help. We must build allies to bring you to your rightful crown."

"But I do not want it," Lotus said.

Master Blade put his hands on her shoulders, looked into her eyes, and said, "My dear Lotus, the country is in need of the wisdom of the lotus. *You* are that Lotus! The evil Queen Teraw will stop at nothing to destroy you now. She rules using the cold force to influence with fear."

"I can do much more to teach you both; to help prepare you for what is to come," Master Talon said.

Brax looked at Lotus and said, "I worry about your safety, even more so now that I know you are the rightful queen. This puts your life in danger. More challenges will surely come."

"Brax, we will both learn from Master Talon, and meet the challenges ahead together. Our love will be our strength, not our weakness. We will go and find the help my father mentioned," Lotus promised.

"Will you go with us, Master Talon?" Brax asked.

"I will go with you as counsel and teacher," Master Talon declared with a humble smile.

And so, the journey began. To be continued in Jade Chi Do, Book 2 - The 8 Infinities of Direction.

To be the first to get this book go to: **www.jadechido.info**